Diagnostic Radiology

FIFTH EDITION

SINGLE BEST ANSWER MCQs

Commissioning Editor: Michael Houston
Development Editor: Alexandra Mortimer
Project Manager: Shereen Jameel
Design: Kirsteen Wright
Marketing Managers (UK/USA): Ria Timmerman, William Veltre

Grainger & Allison's
Diagnostic Radiology
FIFTH EDITION
SINGLE BEST ANSWER MCQs

Andrew S. McQueen, MRCP FRCR
Specialist Registrar, Radiology, Newcastle upon Tyne

Lee A. Grant, MRCS FRCR
Specialist Registrar, Radiology, Cambridge

Jennifer L. Findlay, MRCS
Specialist Registrar, Radiology, Mersey

Sheetal Sharma, MRCP FRCR
Specialist Registrar, Radiology, Newcastle upon Tyne

Vivek Shrivastava, MRCSEd MD
Specialist Registrar, Radiology, Newcastle upon Tyne

Scott M. M. McDonald, MRCSEd FRCR
Specialist Registrar, Radiology, Cambridge

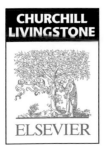

CHURCHILL
LIVINGSTONE

ELSEVIER

CHURCHILL LIVINGSTONE
ELSEVIER

© 2009, Elsevier Limited. All rights reserved.

First published 2009

The right of Andrew S. McQueen, Lee A. Grant, Jennifer L. Findlay, Sheetal Sharma, Vivek Shrivastava and Scott M. M. McDonald to be identified as authors of this work has been asserted by them in accordance with the Copyright, Designs and Patents Act 1988.

978-0-7020-3149-6

Reprinted 2009, 2010

British Library Cataloguing in Publication Data
A catalogue record for this book is available from the British Library

Library of Congress Cataloging in Publication Data
A catalog record for this book is available from the Library of Congress

Notice
Medical knowledge is constantly changing. Standard safety precautions must be followed, but as new research and clinical experience broaden our knowledge, changes in treatment and drug therapy may become necessary or appropriate. Readers are advised to check the most current product information provided by the manufacturer of each drug to be administered to verify the recommended dose, the method and duration of administration, and contraindications. It is the responsibility of the practitioner, relying on experience and knowledge of the patient, to determine dosages and the best treatment for each individual patient. Neither the Publisher nor the authors assume any liability for any injury and/or damage to persons or property arising from this publication.

The Publisher

ELSEVIER your source for books, journals and multimedia in the health sciences
www.elsevierhealth.com

Working together to grow libraries in developing countries

www.elsevier.com | www.bookaid.org | www.sabre.org

ELSEVIER   BOOK AID International   Sabre Foundation

The Publisher's policy is to use paper manufactured from sustainable forests

Printed in China
Last digit is the print number: 9 8 7 6 5 4 3

CONTENTS

Foreword   vii

Preface   ix

Dedication   xi

Acknowledgements   xiii

List of Commonly Used Abbreviations   xv

Module 1: Cardiothoracic and Vascular   **1**

Questions   1

Answers   52

Module 2: Musculoskeletal and Trauma   **79**

Questions   79

Answers   120

Module 3: Gastrointestinal   **137**

Questions   137

Answers   189

Module 4: Genitourinary, Adrenal, Obstetric &
Gynaecology and Breast   **215**

Questions   215

Answers   257

Module 5: Paediatrics   **277**

Questions   277

Answers   318

Module 6: Central Nervous and Head & Neck   **337**

Questions   337

Answers   378

FOREWORD

This Multiple Choice Question book, largely based on facts within the recent fifth edition of *Diagnostic Radiology*, is timely. It is one of the first radiology MCQ book targeted for the FRCR to use the "best of five" options, which are now deemed to be a fairer MCQ test than those where each statement is true or false. Thus this book fully conforms to the style of modern professional postgraduate radiological examinations such as the FRCR in the UK.

The various authors are to be congratulated on achieving a relatively uniform style and providing realistic "negative" suggestions. They have assembled a spread of topics in the various sub-specialties which match the current distribution of FRCR Part II MCQ examination questions. They have also avoided using too much jargon and slang nomenclature which is, sadly, becoming widespread nowadays.

This book will provide reassurance and practice for FRCR candidates and others approaching postgraduate professional examinations. It should also be salutary for more senior radiologists who may be questioning their own factual knowledge base in these days of increasing accreditation legislation.

Andy Adam and Adrian Dixon
On behalf of the editors of Diagnostic Radiology
(Adam, Dixon, Grainger and Allison)
2009

PREFACE

The Final Fellowship of the Royal College of Radiologists (FRCR) Part A Examination comprises six modules, covering the full spectrum of clinical radiology. The fifth edition of *Grainger & Allison's Diagnostic Radiology* is structured to reflect the modular nature of this examination and is a core textbook for revision and preparation. This new edition contains established FRCR exam topics as well as recent imaging developments likely to feature in the forthcoming examinations. In 2008, the Royal College of Radiologists announced proposals to replace the negatively marked true/false format of the Final Part A examination with a new Single Best Answer (SBA) question style. Candidates are required to select a single correct answer from a number of choices and marks are no longer deducted for a wrong answer. This change in question format will significantly alter the nature of the FRCR 2A examination and the revision methods used by candidates. Answering large numbers of true/false questions is no longer essential for developing good FRCR 2A exam technique.

This book contains only SBA questions, drawn primarily from the fifth edition of *Grainger & Allison* and also from widely used radiology textbooks and journals. Each question comprises a short vignette containing clinical and/or imaging findings and the candidate is asked to select the best answer from a list of five options. The answer is accompanied by the full question reference, to enable the candidate to consolidate their knowledge.

We hope that this book will be a comprehensive and well-referenced resource for FRCR 2A candidates and we wish the reader every success!

DEDICATION

This book is dedicated to our families, with gratitude for their love and support.

ACKNOWLEDGEMENTS

The authors wish to thank Professor Adrian Dixon, who generously gave up his time to offer advice and guidance during the preparation of this book, and Dr Liam McKnight, who kindly gave us the benefit of his expertise in question design. We are indebted to Michael Houston for his astute guidance and for enabling our concept of a revision book to become a reality. We also wish to thank Alexandra Mortimer, Shereen Jameel and Charles Lauder for their skill and dedication in shaping our manuscript into the finished work.

LIST OF COMMONLY USED ABBREVIATIONS

^{18}FDG	^{18} fluorodeoxyglucose
μL	Microlitres
ACL	Anterior cruciate ligament
AP	Anteroposterior
CF	Cystic fibrosis
CMV	Cytomegalovirus
CNS	Central nervous system
CRP	C reactive protein
CSF	Cerebrospinal fluid
CT	Computed tomography
CTPA	Computed tomography pulmonary angiogram
CXR	Chest radiograph
DMSA	Dimercaptosuccinic acid
DTPA	Diethylene triamine pentaacetic acid
DWI	Diffusion weighted imaging
ECG	Electrocardiogram
ERCP	Endoscopic retrograde cholangiopancreatography
ESR	Erythrocyte sedimentation rate
FLAIR	Fluid attenuated inversion recovery
GCS	Glasgow coma scale
GIST	Gastrointestinal stromal tumour
GP	General practitioner
Hb	Haemoglobin
HCC	Hepatocellular carcinoma
HIV	Human immunodeficiency virus
HRCT	High resolution computed tomography

HU	Hounsfield Units
ITU	Intensive Therapy Unit
IV	Intravenous
IVU	Intravenous urogram
LFTs	Liver function tests
MAG3	Mercaptoacetyltriglycine
MCPJ	Metacarpophalangeal joint
MCUG	Micturating cystourethrogram
MRCP	Magnetic resonance cholangiopancreatography
MRI	Magnetic resonance imaging
NAI	Nonaccidental injury
NG	Nasogastric
PA	Posteroanterior
PCL	Posterior cruciate ligament
PCP	Pneumocystis carinii pneumonia
PET	Positron emission tomography
SLE	Systemic lupus erythematosus
STIR	Short tau inversion recovery
Tc-99m	Technetium 99m
T1w	T1 weighted
T2w	T2 weighted
US	Ultrasound

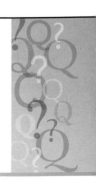

Cardiothoracic and Vascular

QUESTIONS

QUESTION 1

A 30-year-old man presents to his GP with a cough and increasing shortness of breath. A chest radiograph (CXR) reveals the presence of symmetrical hilar masses. These masses have a lobulated and well-defined outline with some fine peripheral calcification. The lesions do not appear cystic or contain any fat. The only occupational exposure of note is that the patient keeps birds in his house. Which is the most likely diagnosis?

A Mature mediastinal teratoma
B Primary tuberculosis
C Sarcoidosis
D Silicosis
E Untreated lymphoma

Answer on page 52

QUESTION 2

A 40-year-old woman has been admitted to the Intensive Therapy Unit (ITU) with severe pancreatitis. She is currently being ventilated but has worsening respiratory failure, refractory to oxygen therapy. In addition, she has a normal capillary wedge pressure. Which of the following is the most likely radiological feature on portable CXR?

A Cardiomegaly
B Mediastinal lymphadenopathy
C Patchy peripheral airspace opacification
D Pleural effusions
E Well-defined lobar airspace opacification

Answer on page 52

QUESTION 3

A 25-year-old asthmatic man is referred to the chest outpatient clinic with a fever, cough and shortness of breath. A course of antibiotics has not improved his symptoms. Investigations performed in the clinic include a positive skin test for *Aspergillus fumigatus* and an elevated serum IgE. The patient is known to be immunocompetent with no previous history of sarcoidosis or tuberculosis. Which one of the following are the most likely high-resolution CT (HRCT) findings?

A A lower lobe predominance
B An air crescent sign
C Central bronchiectasis
D The halo sign
E Wedge-shaped peripheral infarcts

Answer on page 53

QUESTION 4

An 80-year-old lifelong male smoker presents with a cough and wheeze. A CXR demonstrates right middle lobe airspace opacification with bulging of the central oblique and horizontal fissures. The radiographic appearances fail to resolve 4 weeks later, after an appropriate course of antibiotics. CT evaluation demonstrates a large cavitating centrally placed mass. Which one of the following diagnoses is the most likely?

A Adenocarcinoma
B Large cell carcinoma
C Lymphoma
D Small cell carcinoma
E Squamous cell carcinoma

Answer on page 53

QUESTION 5

You are reviewing a contrast-enhanced CT chest for a suspected central bronchogenic carcinoma of the lung. You determine that the tumour is greater than 3 cm in its longest dimension, invades the mediastinal pleura but does not invade any mediastinal structures. There is an associated pleural effusion but you are informed by the clinical team that multiple cytopathological examinations reveal no tumour cells. What would be your proposed T staging?

A TX
B T1
C T2
D T3
E T4

Answer on page 53

QUESTION 6

A 70-year-old man recently underwent a laparoscopic prostatectomy. He now presents to the Emergency Department complaining of shortness of breath, pleuritic chest pain and haemoptysis. D-dimer levels were measured and found to be significantly elevated. A CXR is performed as part of the initial set of investigations. Which one of the following is the most likely CXR finding?

A A normal chest radiograph

B Linear atelectasis

C Localised peripheral oligaemia

D Peripheral airspace opacification

E Pleural effusion

Answer on page 53

QUESTION 7

A 30-year-old male nonsmoker presents to his GP with a three-month history of intermittent episodes of cough and wheeze. Initially diagnosed as having asthma, the patient was found to be α1-antitrypsin deficient after mentioning that several relatives have had similar problems in the past. As part of the subsequent investigations, an HRCT chest was performed. Which finding is most consistent with this clinical scenario?

A Low attenuation regions with a lower lobe predominance

B Low attenuation regions with an upper lobe predominance

C Pleural effusion

D Spontaneous pneumothorax

E Subpleural low attenuation areas

Answer on page 54

QUESTION 8

A 16-year-old man has been sent for a CXR by his GP. He has had a chronic cough for 3 months and the GP is concerned that there may be an underlying pneumonia. Having reviewed the film and decided that this is not the case, you note the presence of a unilateral hypertransradiant hemithorax. Which of the following causes would not be in your differential diagnosis?

A MacLeod's syndrome

B Poland's syndrome

C Poliomyelitis

D Pulmonary agenesis and hypoplasia

E Pulmonary embolus

Answer on page 54

QUESTION 9

An 80-year-old man presents to the Emergency Department chronically short of breath. On examination, there is dullness at the left lung base and a CXR reveals loss of the left costophrenic angle. An ultrasound is performed and demonstrates a pleural effusion with no internal echoes. Diagnostic aspiration reveals that the pleural fluid has a protein concentration of 15 g/L. Which one of the following would be the most likely cause?

A Cardiac failure

B Collagen vascular diseases

C Infection

D Malignancy

E Pulmonary infarction

Answer on page 54

QUESTION 10

A young woman with Turner's syndrome is found to be hypertensive. On examination, her femoral pulses are delayed, relative to the carotid pulses. In addition there is a mid to late systolic murmur. Which one of the following is the most likely radiological finding?

A An '8' sign due to modelling deformities of the major thoracic vessels
B An enlarged external mammary artery on a lateral plain chest radiograph
C Elevated left ventricular apex
D Rib notching affecting all ribs
E Superior rib notching

Answer on page 55

QUESTION 11

A 50-year-old man undergoes a routine preoperative CXR. The reporting radiologist notes that the heart is shifted to the left, the right heart border is indistinct and there is a steep inferior slope of the anterior ribs. Which one of the following syndromes may be associated with these findings?

A Churg Strauss syndrome
B Eisenmenger's syndrome
C MacLeod's syndrome
D Marfan's syndrome
E Swyer James syndrome

Answer on page 55

QUESTION 12

A 60-year-old man with Hodgkin's disease and hypertension complains of shortness of breath. He attends the Radiology Department for a CXR and it is noted that he has bilateral pleural effusions. No lung parenchymal abnormality is identified and a recent transthoracic echocardiogram was normal. It is clinically suspected that the pleural effusions may have been caused by one of the drugs he is currently taking. Which one of his drug treatments is the most likely to have caused the pleural effusions?

A Amoxycillin

B Bleomycin

C Frusemide

D Lisinopril

E Propranolol

Answer on page 55

QUESTION 13

A young man is involved in a road traffic accident and complains of pleuritic chest pain and shortness of breath. An initial supine CXR performed in the Emergency Department demonstrates several left-sided posterior rib fractures. There is also the suspicion that a pneumothorax is present. Once stabilised, the patient attends the Radiology Department for an erect PA chest radiograph. Which one of the following signs not seen on the initial supine film will now predominate?

A A deep left costophrenic recess laterally

B Left apical transradiancy and pleural line

C Undue clarity of the left mediastinal border

D Unilateral left lung transradiancy

E Visualisation of the undersurface of the heart

Answer on page 55

QUESTION 14

A 60-year-old man presents to his GP with a cough, fever, dyspnoea and some chest pain. He also complains of painful wrists and hands which are worse at night. A CXR demonstrated a pleural-based left chest wall mass with a well-demarcated and slightly lobulated contour. No rib destruction is evident. A subsequent CT confirmed these findings with the mass demonstrating slightly heterogeneous enhancement after contrast administration. No pleural effusion was seen. Which one of the following is the most likely diagnosis?

A Empyema

B Localised mesothelioma

C Pleural extension of a lung tumour

D Pleural metastasis

E Subpleural lipoma

Answer on page 56

QUESTION 15

A previously fit and well 30-year-old woman undergoes a CT pulmonary angiogram (CTPA) for suspected acute pulmonary embolism. The CTPA excludes a pulmonary embolism but an incidental mediastinal mass is noted. This solitary mediastinal mass is seen inferior to the carina with displacement of the carina anteriorly and the oesophagus displaced posteriorly. The contents of the lesion are of uniform attenuation 0 Hounsfield Units (HU). Prior to this admission the patient had not reported any symptoms of note. What is the most likely diagnosis?

A Bronchogenic cyst

B Mediastinal pancreatic pseudocyst

C Neurenteric cyst

D Neurogenic tumour

E Oesophageal duplication cyst

Answer on page 56

QUESTION 16

A 40-year-old woman has a previous history of histoplasmosis. She undergoes a chest CT which demonstrates confluent soft tissue infiltration throughout the mediastinum. Tissue biopsy determines a diagnosis of fibrosing mediastinitis subsequent to the histoplasmosis infection. Which one of the following complications would be the most common to occur?

A Oesophageal obstruction

B Pulmonary artery obstruction

C Pulmonary venous obstruction

D Superior vena cava obstruction

E Tracheal obstruction

Answer on page 56

QUESTION 17

A 25-year-old man has a CXR (PA and lateral) performed for a chronic cough. This demonstrates a mass projected anterior to the ascending aorta and a contrast-enhanced CT chest is performed. There are no associated clinical syndromes (such as myasthenia gravis) and no CT features to suggest a thymic mass or germ cell tumour. What additional CT finding is most likely to suggest a diagnosis of lymphangioma?

A Bone destruction

B Multiple cystic spaces

C Narrow contact with the ascending aorta

D Retrosternal extension

E Uniform fat attenuation

Answer on page 56

QUESTION 18

A 27-year-old, previously fit and well man presents to his GP with a short history of pyrexia, cough and haemoptysis. He has never previously been admitted to hospital. Sputum culture has grown *Streptococcus pneumoniae*. What is the most likely chest radiograph finding?

A Bronchopneumonia
B Cavitation
C Empyema
D Large pleural effusion
E Lobar consolidation

Answer on page 57

QUESTION 19

An 80-year-old man has been admitted to hospital with shortness of breath and a productive, purulent cough. A CXR reveals left lower lobe consolidation. Which additional radiological finding is most likely to suggest a diagnosis of *Klebsiella pneumoniae* rather than *Legionella pneumophila*?

A Bulging fissures
B Mediastinal lymphadenopathy
C Pleural effusion
D Pneumothorax
E Septal thickening

Answer on page 57

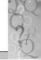

QUESTION 20

A 7-year-old girl, who has recently migrated to this country from India, presents with a productive cough, fever, night sweats and weight loss. A CXR demonstrates marked consolidation in the right upper lobe. Sputum cytology reveals the presence of acid fast bacilli. What additional radiological finding is most likely to suggest a diagnosis of current primary tuberculosis as opposed to post-primary tuberculosis?

A Cavitation
B Mediastinal lymphadenopathy
C Multifocal lesions
D Ranke complex
E Rasmussen aneurysm

Answer on page 57

QUESTION 21

A 30-year-old male engineer has recently returned from North America having inspected a number of construction sites. He develops flu-like symptoms and a CXR reveals the presence of a solitary well-defined nodule. What additional finding would make a diagnosis of *Histoplasmosis* infection more likely, rather than *Cryptococcus* infection?

A Air bronchograms
B Cavitation
C Central calcification
D Lymphadenopathy
E Pleural effusion

Answer on page 57

QUESTION 22

A 35-year-old man complains of a cough and is sent for a CXR by his GP. This demonstrates a solitary cystic structure within the left lower lobe, measuring approximately 6 cm in diameter. The peripheral aspect of the cystic structure lies in contact with the chest wall and appears slightly flattened. Within this structure there appears to be a floating membrane. What is the most likely diagnosis?

A Aspergillosis

B Coccidioidomycosis

C Hydatid disease

D *Mycoplasma pneumoniae*

E Tuberculosis

Answer on page 58

QUESTION 23

A 30-year-old man is HIV positive with a most recent CD4 count = 100 cells/μL. He presents to the infectious diseases team with a cough, dyspnoea and general malaise. A CXR demonstrates bilateral, diffuse, medium-sized reticular opacities. An air-filled parenchymal cavity (pneumatocoele) is seen, but there is an absence of either mediastinal lymphadenopathy or a pleural effusion. What is the most likely underlying opportunistic infection?

A *Streptococcus pneumoniae*

B *Cryptococcus neoformans*

C *Cytomegalovirus*

D *Mycobacterium avium* complex

E *Pneumocystis carinii*

Answer on page 58

QUESTION 24

A 38-year-old man is referred to a chest physician for evaluation of a chronic productive cough. Over the past 10 years he has experienced increased expectoration of mucoid sputum that became purulent during infective exacerbations. On plain radiography the trachea had a corrugated outline. CT evaluation revealed dilatation of the trachea and mainstream bronchi. Which one of the following is the most likely diagnosis?

A Amyloidosis

B Mounier-Kuhn disease

C Relapsing polychondritis

D Tracheal leiomyoma

E Wegener's granulomatosis

Answer on page 58

QUESTION 25

A 20-year-old woman with cystic fibrosis undergoes an HRCT chest as a result of worsening respiratory function. Nontapering, thickened bronchi are easily seen within 1 cm of the costal pleura. The internal bronchial diameter is greater than that of the adjacent pulmonary artery and the bronchial lumen has assumed a beaded configuration. Whilst there are V- and Y-shaped densities, the 'tree in bud' sign and mosaic perfusion are not seen. What is the most likely diagnosis?

A Bronchiolitis

B Cylindrical bronchiectasis

C Cystic bronchiectasis

D Infective consolidation

E Varicose bronchiectasis

Answer on page 58

QUESTION 26

A 15-year-old girl has a follow-up CXR and ultrasound scan of her liver. She is known to have had meconium ileus at birth and has subsequently suffered with recurrent chest infections, poor weight gain, loose malodorous stools and multiple gallstones. Which of the following findings is most likely to be present on the CXR?

    A Bronchiectasis with a predominant lower lobe distribution

    B Ground glass opacity

    C In-dwelling venous catheter

    D Pleural effusion

    E Reduced lung volumes

Answer on page 59

QUESTION 27

A 60-year-old woman with rheumatoid arthritis presents with a flu-like illness and nonproductive cough. Her symptoms have not responded to an appropriate course of antibiotics. An HRCT is performed and demonstrates widespread mosaic perfusion. Which additional CT finding would suggest a diagnosis of obliterative bronchiolitis rather than diffuse pulmonary haemorrhage?

    A Increased calibre pulmonary vessels in the hyperattenuated area

    B Increased calibre pulmonary vessels in the hypoattenuated area

    C Normal calibre pulmonary vessels in the hyperattenuated area

    D Reduced calibre pulmonary vessels in the hypoattenuated area

    E Reduced calibre pulmonary vessels in the hyperattenuated area

Answer on page 59

QUESTION 28

A 50-year-old lifelong male smoker has presented to his GP with increasing shortness of breath. A CXR shows that the right atrial border is a little indistinct. On the lateral view there is a triangular density with its apex directed towards the lung hilum. Which one of the following is the most likely diagnosis?

A Left lower lobe collapse

B Left upper lobe collapse

C Right middle lobe collapse

D Right lower lobe collapse

E Right upper lobe collapse

Answer on page 59

QUESTION 29

You are asked to review the CT scan of an elderly female patient who has evidence of left upper lobe collapse on a CXR. On CT, in which one of the following directions will the left upper lobe have collapsed?

A Anteriorly and laterally

B Anteriorly and medially

C Inferiorly and medially

D Posteriorly and medially

E Superiorly and medially

Answer on page 59

QUESTION 30

A previously fit and well 70-year-old man has a routine CXR prior to a left hip replacement. An incidental right hilar mass is noted with associated right middle lobe collapse and bulging of the oblique and horizontal fissures. Cavitation is seen within the mass and mediastinal lymphadenopathy is demonstrated on the subsequent CT examination. No calcification is demonstrated within the mass. What is the most likely diagnosis?

A Arteriovenous malformation

B Aspergilloma

C Empyema

D Sarcoidosis

E Squamous cell carcinoma

Answer on page 60

QUESTION 31

A 50-year-old female patient with Cushing's syndrome presents with a wheeze and nonresolving left lower lobe consolidation. CT reveals a calcified polypoid tumour lying external to the left main bronchus, with a smaller intraluminal component causing partial left lower lobe obstruction. Marked enhancement is seen after the administration of contrast medium. What is the most likely diagnosis?

A Bronchial carcinoid

B Bronchial chondroma

C Bronchial fibroma

D Bronchial haemangioma

E Bronchial hamartoma

Answer on page 60

QUESTION 32

A middle-aged man has recently had a CT abdomen performed for chronic lower left abdominal pain. Whilst mild sigmoid diverticular disease was present, it was also noted that there was significant para-aortic lymphadenopathy. Lymphoma was the suspected diagnosis and a chest CT was performed, prior to biopsy. Which additional CT finding is most likely to suggest a diagnosis of non-Hodgkin's lymphoma rather than Hodgkin's disease?

  A Isolated pulmonary consolidation
  B Paramediastinal interstitial fibrosis
  C Peripheral subpleural masses with a pleural effusion
  D Peripheral subpleural masses without a pleural effusion
  E Pulmonary consolidation with mediastinal lymphadenopathy

Answer on page 60

QUESTION 33

A confused 70-year-old man with a history of cough and some shortness of breath attends your Radiology Department for a CXR. It is noted that there are multiple discrete, spherical and well-defined pulmonary nodules with a peripheral distribution. Some calcification is noted within some of these nodules but cavitation is not evident. The accompanying nurse from the care home tells you that he has a 'growth' somewhere but is not sure what this is. What is the most likely primary tumour?

  A Adenocarcinoma of the colon
  B Anaplastic thyroid carcinoma
  C Chondrosarcoma of the femur
  D Invasive ductal carcinoma of the breast
  E Squamous cell carcinoma of the oesophagus

Answer on page 60

QUESTION 34

A previously fit and well 50-year-old man presents with progressive dyspnoea for one year. On CXR, there are bilateral, peripheral reticular opacities seen at the lung bases. On HRCT chest, there is a subpleural basal reticular pattern with areas of honeycomb change seen. Which one of the following is the most likely diagnosis?

A Acute interstitial pneumonia (AIP)

B Cryptogenic organising pneumonia (COP)

C Desquamative interstitial pneumonia (DIP)

D Nonspecific interstitial pneumonia (NSIP)

E Usual interstitial pneumonia (UIP)

Answer on page 61

QUESTION 35

A 50-year-old woman with rheumatoid arthritis undergoes an HRCT chest following a gradual increase in shortness of breath. Interstitial inflammation and fibrosis is noted. What additional finding is most likely to suggest a diagnosis of NSIP rather than UIP?

A Honeycombing

B Irregular changes over time

C Mediastinal lymphadenopathy

D Prominent ground glass attenuation

E Upper lobe predominance

Answer on page 61

QUESTION 36

A 20-year-old woman presents with a dry cough and dyspnoea. A CXR has been performed and demonstrates bilateral hilar lymphadenopathy with bilateral well-defined 3 mm parenchymal nodules. The diagnosis is most likely to be?

A Stage 0 Sarcoidosis

B Stage 1 Sarcoidosis

C Stage 2 Sarcoidosis

D Stage 3 Sarcoidosis

E Stage 4 Sarcoidosis

Answer on page 61

QUESTION 37

A 30-year-old woman has had an HRCT as a result of increasing shortness of breath. As well as mediastinal lymphadenopathy, it demonstrates well-defined nodular opacities (approximately 3 mm in diameter) found subpleurally and along the bronchovascular bundles. There is a predominantly mid to upper zone distribution with some air trapping demonstrated. Which one of the following is the most likely diagnosis?

A Acute extrinsic allergic alveolitis

B Langerhans cell histiocytosis

C Lymphangioleiomyomatosis

D Sarcoidosis

E Usual interstitial pneumonia

Answer on page 61

QUESTION 38

A 30-year-old man has had an HRCT reviewed at your local multidisciplinary team meeting. The HRCT demonstrates ground glass opacification throughout both lungs with a mosaic pattern on expiratory images. Which additional finding would make a diagnosis of extrinsic allergic alveolitis (EAI) more likely than respiratory bronchiolitis–interstitial lung disease (RB-ILD)?

A A normal chest radiograph

B A positive smoking history

C A stable clinical course

D Exposure to paint sprays

E Poorly defined centrilobular nodules

Answer on page 62

QUESTION 39

A 30-year-old patient has presented with a nonproductive cough, fatigue, weight loss and a fever. As a result of an abnormality seen on a CXR, an HRCT chest is performed and demonstrates multiple thin-walled cysts within the lung parenchyma. Which additional finding is most likely to suggest a diagnosis of Langerhans cell histiocytosis (LCH) rather than lymphangioleiomyomatosis?

A A smoking history

B Female sex

C Increased lung volumes

D No zonal predilection

E Pleural effusion

Answer on page 62

QUESTION 40

A 30-year-old woman complains of shortness of breath and a CXR is requested. The request form states 'connective tissue disease' but no further medical history is provided. The CXR demonstrates mild pleural thickening with small, bilateral pleural effusions. Interstitial fibrosis, with some honeycomb formation, is seen within the lower lung zones. In addition there is a single, well-circumscribed 2 cm lesion in the right upper zone, with an area of cavitation seen centrally. Which one of the following connective tissue diseases is the most likely diagnosis?

A Ankylosing spondylitis

B Dermatomyositis

C Rheumatoid arthritis

D Scleroderma

E Systemic lupus erythematosus

Answer on page 62

QUESTION 41

A 30-year-old woman presents with a history of a low grade fever, malaise, anorexia and weight loss. She also reports pleuritic type chest pain. A CXR shows bilateral small pleural effusions with linear band atelectasis at both bases. No other chest abnormality is seen. Which one of the following is the most likely diagnosis?

A Ankylosing spondylitis

B Dermatomyositis

C Rheumatoid arthritis

D Scleroderma

E Systemic lupus erythematosus

Answer on page 62

QUESTION 42

A 40-year-old man presents with rhinitis, sinusitis and otitis media. In addition he has dyspnoea and pleuritic chest pain and has had episodes of haemoptysis. His records indicate that he has had a recent renal biopsy which diagnosed the presence of focal necrotising glomerulonephritis. Which one of the following is the most likely radiological finding demonstrated on chest CT?

A Lobular mass with feeding and draining vessels
B Mediastinal lymphadenopathy
C Multiple cavitating lung parenchymal nodules
D Parenchymal mass lesion with lobar collapse
E Upper lobe mycetoma

Answer on page 63

QUESTION 43

A 63-year-old man attends the Radiology Department for a CXR.
He presented to his GP with a chronic cough and breathlessness and an occupational history of having worked both in a quarry and, later on in his life, as a coal miner. Which one of the following radiographic findings is most likely to suggest a diagnosis of silicosis rather than coal worker's pneumoconiosis (CWP)?

A A predominantly upper lobe distribution of disease
B Eggshell calcification of mediastinal lymph nodes
C Large (greater than 3 mm) lung nodules
D Progressive massive fibrosis
E Small (up to 3 mm) lung nodules

Answer on page 63

QUESTION 44

A 40-year-old former construction worker presents with increasing dyspnoea and purulent sputum production. A CXR demonstrates lobar consolidation and he is treated for community-acquired pneumonia. However, incidental note is made of the presence of pleural plaques, which are assumed to be the result of asbestos exposure. Which one of the following radiological features would be most in keeping with asbestos related pleural plaques?

A Distribution along the anterior chest wall
B Involvement of the parietal pleura
C Mediastinal lymphadenopathy
D Sparing of the diaphragmatic dome
E Sparing of the mediastinal pleura

Answer on page 63

QUESTION 45

A 60 year-old man, with a known history of asbestos exposure, is seen in the chest outpatient clinic with increasing shortness of breath. A CT chest is performed and demonstrates a subpleural mass in the right lower lobe with thickening of the adjacent pleura. Which additional radiological finding is most likely to reassure you that this is not a bronchogenic carcinoma?

A An acute angle made by the mass with the surrounding pleura
B 'Comet tail' sign
C Homogeneous contrast enhancement
D The lesion is solitary
E Volume loss in the lower lobe

Answer on page 63

QUESTION 46

A 25-year-old male pedestrian has been hit by a car and is currently being resuscitated in the Emergency Department. He complains of paraesthesia involving his left shoulder. Which one of the following radiological features is the most likely related cause?

A Dislocated left sternoclavicular joint
B Fractured left 2nd rib
C Fractured left humerus
D Left tension pneumothorax
E Right anterior shoulder dislocation

Answer on page 64

QUESTION 47

A 40-year-old male window cleaner has fallen approximately 4 m from his ladder whilst at work. He is currently on a spinal board and being assessed in the resuscitation department of your Emergency Department. He complains of left-sided chest pain and shortness of breath. A CXR demonstrates fractures of the left 3rd, 4th and 5th lateral ribs and there is strong clinical concern of a pneumothorax. If there is a left pneumothorax, which one of the following radiographic signs is most likely to be present?

A A left-sided haemothorax
B An abnormally deep left costophrenic sulcus
C Left upper lobe pulmonary contusion
D Mediastinal shift towards the left
E Visible visceral pleura with absent lung markings peripherally

Answer on page 64

QUESTION 48

A 27-year-old man has been involved in a high-speed road traffic accident. There is significant diagonal bruising over the abdomen, due to the wearing of a seat belt. He is haemodynamically stable, but complains of severe abdominal pain and a CT of the chest and abdomen is performed. Which one of the following radiographic signs on a CXR would be most likely to suggest a right-sided diaphragmatic injury?

A A nasogastric tube coiled within the left hemithorax

B A right pleural effusion

C Elevated left hemidiaphragm

D Hollow viscera seen within the chest

E Mediastinal shift towards the left

Answer on page 64

QUESTION 49

A 42-year-old woman has been involved in a road traffic accident, having lost control of her car and collided with a lorry. She complains of left-sided chest and abdominal pain and was initially hypotensive, but has responded to fluid resuscitation. CT examination has demonstrated the presence of left-sided rib fractures, a left haemothorax and a splenic laceration. Which one of the following CT signs is least likely to be associated with rupture of the left hemidiaphragm?

A Discontinuity of the left hemidiaphragm

B Herniation of the colon into the chest

C The 'collar sign'

D The 'dependent viscera sign'

E The 'target sign'

Answer on page 64

QUESTION 50

A 30-year-old warehouse employee has been admitted to the Emergency Department, having been crushed between a reversing lorry and a wall. A supine CXR demonstrates a pneumomediastinum and a right-sided pneumothorax that has not responded to the insertion of an appropriately sited chest drain. The right lung is seen to sag towards the floor of the right hemithorax. Which one of the following is the most likely diagnosis?

A Flail chest

B Pneumopericardium

C Ruptured oesophagus

D Tracheobronchial rupture

E Traumatic aortic rupture

Answer on page 65

QUESTION 51

A 60-year-old female driver lost control of her car on black ice and hit a tree at approximately 60 miles per hour. Following resuscitation in the Emergency Department, she is found to have serious head and limb injuries and complains of upper thoracic back pain. Which one of the following radiographic signs would make you most suspicious for the presence of a traumatic aortic rupture?

A A left apical pleural cap

B A mediastinum more than 5 cm wide

C A right apical pleural cap

D Deviation of the trachea to the left

E Widening of the left paratracheal stripe

Answer on page 65

QUESTION 52

A 30-year-old man with a history of heavy alcohol abuse has been admitted to ITU with severe acute pancreatitis. He is currently ventilated and afebrile, but has worsening respiratory failure, diminished pulmonary compliance and a normal capillary wedge pressure. The clinical team suspect a diagnosis of acute respiratory distress syndrome. Which one of the following radiographic signs would you not expect to see in acute respiratory distress syndrome (ARDS)?

A Complete resolution of the lung abnormality

B Diffuse ground glass opacities with a bilateral distribution

C Diffuse ground glass opacities with a peripheral distribution

D Diffuse ground glass opacities with air bronchograms

E Pleural effusions on plain supine radiography

Answer on page 65

QUESTION 53

An elderly alcoholic man has been admitted to hospital having been found unconscious at home by a neighbour. A CT head has found no cause for his collapse and he is admitted to a medical ward. Twelve hours later, he is found to be increasingly breathless and hypoxic and a CXR is performed. Which one of the following findings is most likely to suggest aspiration?

A A 48-hour delay in the development of radiographic infiltrates following aspiration

B Bilateral pleural effusions

C Pulmonary infiltrates with an upper lobe predominance

D Regression of radiographic pulmonary changes after 72 hours

E Well-defined pulmonary infiltrates

Answer on page 65

QUESTION 54

A middle-aged woman is currently ventilated on ITU following a major episode of sepsis and multiorgan failure. Her respiratory function is declining and a mobile CXR shows patchy pulmonary infiltrates within both lungs. A diagnosis of pulmonary oedema is suspected. Which one of the following radiological findings is most likely to suggest a diagnosis of noncardiac rather than cardiogenic pulmonary oedema?

A Cardiomegaly

B Central perihilar airspace opacification

C Interstitial lines

D Peribronchial cuffing

E Pleural effusions

Answer on page 66

QUESTION 55

A number of patients on ITU have had CXRs performed as part of their daily investigations. You have been asked to comment on the positioning of various lines and tubes. Which one of the following line/tube tip locations corresponds with the ideal position?

A Central venous pressure catheter within the inferior vena cava

B Endotracheal tube 1 cm above the carina

C Nasogastric tube within the lower oesophagus

D Peripherally inserted central line catheter within the brachiocephalic vein

E Swan-Ganz catheter 5 cm distal to the pulmonary arterial bifurcation

Answer on page 66

QUESTION 56

A 25-year-old man with severe cystic fibrosis has just undergone a double lung transplant. On day 9 postoperatively, he develops diffuse, bilateral airspace opacities, interstitial lines and pleural effusions. There are no other signs to suggest that this is due to cardiac failure. Which one of the following is the most likely diagnosis?

A Acute rejection
B Bronchial stenosis
C Obliterative bronchiolitis
D Post-transplantation lymphoproliferative disease (PTLD)
E Reperfusion oedema

Answer on page 66

QUESTION 57

A 47-year-old man complains of gradually increasing shortness of breath, a dry cough and weight loss. His chest physician is concerned about the possibility of alveolar proteinosis and is particularly keen to exclude the presence of ground glass opacification on his recently performed HRCT examination. After an initial review there are no obvious abnormalities. Which one of the following radiological signs may help diagnose the presence of subtle ground glass opacification?

A The 'Black Bronchus' sign
B The 'Deep Sulcus' sign
C The 'Sail' sign
D The 'Westermark' sign
E The 'V sign of Naclerio'

Answer on page 66

QUESTION 58

A 70-year-old woman complains of progressive dyspnoea. She undergoes an HRCT of the chest and this demonstrates interstitial thickening at the lung bases. Which additional radiological finding would suggest a diagnosis of pulmonary fibrosis rather than congestive heart failure?

A Honeycomb destruction
B Peribronchial cuffing
C Pleural effusion
D Rapid resolution on subsequent chest radiographs
E Upper lobe blood diversion

Answer on page 67

QUESTION 59

A 61-year-old woman attends the Emergency Department complaining of increasingly severe shortness of breath. A CXR shows bilateral airspace opacification with a predominantly central distribution. In addition, there are thickened interlobular septa seen in the subpleural lung and the walls of the visible airways appear thickened and a little indistinct. Which one of the following is the most likely diagnosis?

A Cystic bronchiectasis
B Idiopathic pulmonary fibrosis
C Pulmonary infarct
D Pulmonary lobar collapse
E Pulmonary oedema

Answer on page 67

QUESTION 60

A 43-year-old man presents with a cough, fever and two episodes of haemoptysis. As a result of changes seen on a CXR, a CT chest has been performed. This demonstrates multiple nodules throughout both lungs with no zonal predilection. Cavitation is seen in some of the nodules and others have areas of ground glass opacification surrounding them. Which one of the following is the most likely diagnosis?

A Metastatic lung disease

B Multiple pulmonary infarcts

C Rheumatoid lung nodules

D Sarcoidosis

E Wegener's granulomatosis

Answer on page 67

QUESTION 61

A 22-year-old man presents with a nonproductive cough and exertional dyspnoea, with intermittent chest pain and haemoptysis. On examination, there are inspiratory crackles and digital clubbing and a CXR reveals bilateral, symmetrical airspace opacification. Which additional finding on HRCT is most likely to suggest a diagnosis of alveolar proteinosis rather than eosinophilic lung disease?

A A 'crazy-paving' pattern of the lung parenchyma

B Airway opacification with a peripheral predilection

C Mediastinal lymphadenopathy

D Pleural effusion

E Rapid resolution with steroid therapy

Answer on page 67

QUESTION 62

A 70-year-old man has had a routine CXR prior to an elective total hip replacement. It is noted that the heart is enlarged (the cardiothoracic ratio exceeds 50%). What is the most likely underlying pathology?

A Atrial enlargement

B Cardiac myxoma

C Constrictive pericarditis

D Pericardial effusion

E Ventricular enlargement

Answer on page 68

QUESTION 63

A 50-year-old woman presents with increasing dyspnoea and orthopnoea. There is a significant past history of breast cancer treated with surgery and radiotherapy. Posterior to anterior (PA) and lateral CXRs are performed and demonstrate that the heart size is at the upper limit of normal. Which additional finding is most likely to suggest a diagnosis of constrictive pericarditis rather than acute pericarditis?

A Bilateral hilar overlay

B Effacement of the normal cardiac borders

C Epicardial fat pad sign

D Filling in of the retrosternal space

E Pericardial calcification

Answer on page 68

QUESTION 64

A 45-year-old man presents to the Emergency Department with increasing shortness of breath following a long-haul flight. A CTPA is performed and excludes the presence of a pulmonary embolus. However, cardiac abnormalities are noted and further questioning reveals that the patient had rheumatic fever as a child. Which additional radiological finding is most likely to suggest a diagnosis of rheumatic mitral regurgitation rather than rheumatic mitral stenosis?

A Alveolar pulmonary oedema
B Enlarged left atrial appendage
C Enlarged left atrium
D Left ventricular enlargement
E Tricuspid regurgitation

Answer on page 68

QUESTION 65

A 52-year-old man presents with a long history of right iliac fossa pain, intermittent diarrhoea and weight loss. He has also experienced episodes of flushing, wheezing and dyspnoea. A CT abdomen reveals a calcified mesenteric mass with retraction of the surrounding tissues. There is evidence of multiple liver metastases and a diagnosis of metastatic carcinoid is made. On cardiac MRI, which one of the following is the most likely radiological finding?

A Aortic regurgitation
B Mitral regurgitation
C Mitral stenosis
D Tricuspid regurgitation
E Tricuspid stenosis

Answer on page 68

QUESTION 66

A 30-year-old woman presents with a history of increasing fatigue, breathlessness, chest pain and syncope. A CXR demonstrates aortic valve calcification and a rounded cardiac apex suggestive of left ventricular hypertrophy. Which additional radiological finding is most likely to suggest a diagnosis of rheumatic aortic stenosis rather than calcific aortic stenosis?

A Cardiac dilatation

B Coronary artery disease

C Left atrial enlargement

D Gross aortic calcification

E Post stenotic aortic dilatation

Answer on page 69

QUESTION 67

A 20-year-old professional footballer complains of dyspnoea and palpitations with occasional episodes of syncope. He has had an echocardiogram at another hospital which has raised the possibility of hypertrophic cardiomyopathy. Which one of the following is the most likely MRI finding?

A Dilated left ventricle

B Mitral regurgitation

C Rapid early diastolic ventricular filling

D Reduced cardiac contractility

E Systolic anterior motion of the mitral valve

Answer on page 69

QUESTION 68

A young man presents with generalised fatigue, dyspnoea and episodes of chest pain. A transthoracic echocardiogram has raised the possibility of a cardiac tumour. Which one of the following signs on CT is least likely to be seen with a malignant cardiac neoplasm?

A Cardiac wall destruction

B Involvement of more than one cardiac chamber

C Narrow attachment to the cardiac wall

D Pericardial invasion

E Pulmonary vein extension

Answer on page 69

QUESTION 69

A 72-year-old woman is seen by her GP with a history of palpitations and congestive cardiac failure. A transthoracic echocardiogram is performed and raises the concern that a cardiac tumour may be present. She attends the radiology department for a cardiac MRI examination. From this list of diagnoses and MRI findings, which one is correct?

A Cardiac angiosarcoma most commonly produces a left ventricular mass.

B Cardiac fibroma most commonly produces right atrial wall enlargement.

C Cardiac lymphoma most commonly produces a focal right atrial mass.

D Cardiac myxoma most commonly produces a left atrial mass.

E Cardiac rhabdomyoma most commonly produces interatrial septal enlargement.

Answer on page 69

QUESTION 70

A 50-year-old man complains of increasing chest pains on exertion. He describes this as a dull crushing pain that radiates to his jaw and his GP refers him for an exercise tolerance test. This demonstrates ischaemic ECG changes with chest pain after minimal exertion. Which radiological finding is most likely to be present?

A Increased wall motion on cardiac MRI

B Left anterior descending artery dilatation on cardiac CT angiogram

C No coronary calcification on cardiac CT

D Normal perfusion on stress cardiac scintigraphy

E Reduced distortion of the tagging grid on cardiac MRI

Answer on page 70

QUESTION 71

A 50-year-old lifelong male smoker has had an acute episode of central crushing chest pain and shortness of breath. ECG and serum cardiac enzyme levels are consistent with an acute myocardial infarction. He undergoes a cardiac MRI for further assessment. Which one of the following is the most likely finding?

A Delayed myocardial enhancement with gadolinium perfusion agents

B Increased patency of a coronary artery on contrast-enhanced MR angiography

C Low myocardial signal on T2w images two days post-infarction

D Normal cardiac wall motion using cine-MR imaging

E Normal myocardial perfusion with first-pass contrast medium MR imaging

Answer on page 70

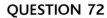

QUESTION 72

A 59-year-old woman complains of shortness of breath, palpitations and dizziness. An ECG demonstrates changes consistent with coronary artery disease and a CT coronary angiogram is performed. Which one of the following is the most likely associated radiological finding?

A A haemodynamically significant stenosis defined as a reduction of at least 30% of luminal diameter

B Absence of flow beyond a stenosis which is pathognomonic for acute arterial occlusion

C An initial increase in the outer diameter of the coronary artery wall

D Calcification of the main pulmonary arteries

E Significant impairment of left ventricular function with an ejection fraction <70%

Answer on page 70

QUESTION 73

A 41-year-old man has previously had a large anterior myocardial infarction. He now presents with increasing shortness of breath on exertion and it is suspected that he has a degree of pulmonary venous hypertension (PVH) due to left ventricular failure. Which one of the following is the most likely radiological finding?

A A fine nodular parenchymal lung pattern if chronic PVH develops

B Kerley A septal lines radiating from the hilum to the pleural surface

C Kerley C septal lines seen at right angles to the pleural surface within the peripheral lower zones

D Lower lobe pulmonary venous blood diversion

E Relative thinning of bronchial wall thickness compared with normal subjects

Answer on page 70

QUESTION 74

A 67-year-old woman presents with a sudden onset of dyspnoea and orthopnoea, following a recent myocardial infarction. Clinical examination reveals a pansystolic murmur with a thrusting apex beat. CXR demonstrates pulmonary oedema with a normal heart size. The suspected diagnosis is severe mitral regurgitation secondary to a ruptured chorda tendinea. Which one of the following signs is associated with this diagnosis?

A Airspace opacification predominantly in a central distribution

B Airspace opacification predominantly in a peripheral distribution

C Airspace opacification predominantly in the left lower zone

D Airspace opacification predominantly in the left upper zone

E Airspace opacification predominantly in the right upper zone

Answer on page 71

QUESTION 75

A 33-year-old woman presents to the Emergency Department with gradually increasing shortness of breath, such that now it is interfering with her daily activities. She has previously been diagnosed with a pulmonary embolus and it is thought that she may have pulmonary arterial hypertension as a result of chronic pulmonary thromboembolic disease. Which one of the following radiological signs is the most likely to be demonstrated?

A A right descending pulmonary artery measuring 10 mm in diameter

B Calcification of the pulmonary arteries

C Lobulated hilar masses

D Peripheral pulmonary arterial branches seen beyond a segmental level

E The diameter of the main pulmonary artery is less than the ascending aorta

Answer on page 71

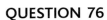

QUESTION 76

Whilst reporting a CXR requested by a GP, you note that the left lung demonstrates reduced pulmonary vascularity relative to the right lung and are undecided as to whether this is an 'apparent' or 'real' finding. Which one of the following conditions is a 'real' cause of uneven pulmonary vascularity?

A MacLeod's syndrome

B Mastectomy

C Patient rotation

D Patient scoliosis

E Poland's syndrome

Answer on page 71

QUESTION 77

A 37-year-old woman presents with episodes of dyspnoea, hypoxia and cyanosis. Initial laboratory investigations are unremarkable and a tuberculin test is negative. On her CXR, there is a lobulated opacity in the left lower lobe with an associated prominent vascular shadow. Inspiratory and expiratory films demonstrate a change in the size of the opacity. What is the most likely diagnosis?

A Pulmonary arteriovenous malformation

B Pulmonary artery pseudoaneurysm

C Pulmonary embolus

D Pulmonary plethora

E Rasmussen aneurysm

Answer on page 71

QUESTION 78

A 50-year-old woman has recently undergone major pelvic surgery. She was previously fit and well but now presents with acute onset of shortness of breath. The clinician suspects a diagnosis of pulmonary embolism and requests a CXR to exclude an alternative cause for the symptoms. Which of the following is the least likely radiological finding if an acute pulmonary embolus is present?

A Central pulmonary arterial enlargement

B Hampton's hump

C Normal chest radiograph

D Small pleural effusion

E Westermark's sign

Answer on page 72

QUESTION 79

A 57-year-old man presents with shortness of breath and a cough. A CXR is normal and ventilation perfusion imaging using Tc-99m microaggregate albumin (MAA) and ^{81m}Kr is performed. Which one of the following diagnoses is unlikely to demonstrate a reversed mismatch ventilation and perfusion defect?

A Chronic obstructive pulmonary disease (COPD)

B Lobar collapse

C Pleural effusion

D Pulmonary consolidation

E Pulmonary embolism

Answer on page 72

QUESTION 80

A 71-year-old man has collapsed at home, having complained of pleuritic chest pain and shortness of breath. He has had similar episodes in the past caused by pulmonary emboli. What finding on review of his CTPA would be consistent with a diagnosis of acute rather than chronic pulmonary embolic disease?

A Calcified pulmonary arterial thrombus
B Crescentic thrombus adherent to the arterial wall
C Enlarged pulmonary arteries
D Mosaic attenuation of the lung parenchyma
E 'Tram track' appearance of a pulmonary artery

Answer on page 72

QUESTION 81

A 73-year-old man presents to his GP with steadily increasing shortness of breath and significant weight loss. His CXR reveals multiple small soft tissue masses throughout both lungs and pulmonary metastases are suspected. Which one of the following statements is true regarding the radiographic appearance of lung metastases?

A Calcification is commonly seen in lung metastases.
B Cavitation is most commonly seen in squamous cell carcinoma metastases.
C They are usually central in distribution.
D They are usually irregular in shape and ill defined.
E The majority are single lesions.

Answer on page 72

QUESTION 82

A male teenager with a known diagnosis of cystic fibrosis (CF) presents with steadily increasing shortness of breath. He is pyrexial and has a cough productive of yellow sputum. A CXR demonstrates longstanding bronchiectatic changes and an HRCT is performed. Which one of the following statements is true regarding HRCT findings in CF?

A Bronchial wall thinning is typically seen.

B Bronchiectasis is present in all patients with advanced CF.

C Lung volume loss is an early finding in CF.

D The earliest lung changes are typically seen in the lower lobes.

E The 'tree-in-bud' sign is a late finding in CF.

Answer on page 73

QUESTION 83

A 35-year-old man presents with increasing shortness of breath, fever and a non productive cough. He is known to be HIV-positive and a recent CD4 count was 110 cells per cubic millimetre. What additional finding is likely to suggest a diagnosis of *Pneumocystis jiroveci (carinii)* rather than tuberculosis?

A A lower lobe predominance

B Bilateral, diffuse, coarse reticulonodular opacities

C Bilateral, diffuse, fine reticular opacities

D Bilateral hilar lymphadenopathy

E Pleural effusions

Answer on page 73

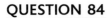

QUESTION 84

A 56-year-old female smoker presents with increasing shortness of breath, fever and a productive cough. Her CXR demonstrates diffuse opacification at the right lung base and treatment is commenced for community-acquired pneumonia. Which additional radiological finding is most likely to suggest a diagnosis of *Streptococcus pneumoniae* rather than *Staphylococcus aureus*?

A Air bronchograms
B Cavitating nodules
C Empyema
D Pleural effusion
E Scattered multifocal opacities

Answer on page 73

QUESTION 85

A 28-year-old woman has had a CXR following the development of a persistent cough. The PA and lateral views demonstrate a significant mediastinal mass. Which one of the following is the correct radiological consideration as you review these films?

A Bronchogenic cysts are usually symptomatic.
B Bronchogenic cysts commonly display calcification of the cyst wall.
C Bronchogenic cysts commonly have a peripheral distribution.
D Neurenteric cysts are usually found in the middle mediastinum.
E Neurenteric cysts are frequently symptomatic.

Answer on page 73

QUESTION 86

A 55-year-old man with a history of uncontrolled hypertension presents with acute, severe chest pain radiating through to his back. A contrast-enhanced CT chest and abdomen (arterial phase) is performed. This confirms the presence of an intimal dissection flap affecting only the descending thoracic aorta (distal to the left subclavian artery) without extension into the abdomen. What is the appropriate radiological classification?

A DeBakey type I

B DeBakey type II

C DeBakey type IIIa

D DeBakey type IIIb

E Stanford type A

Answer on page 74

QUESTION 87

A 21-year-old woman presents with fever, arthralgia and weight loss. A clavicular bruit is detected clinically as well as by diminished upper extremity pulses. Catheter pulmonary and aortic arch angiography is performed and the findings suggest a diagnosis of Takayasu's disease. Which one of the following angiographic findings is most likely to have been present?

A Aortic dissection

B Intercostal collateral development

C Pseudoaneurysm development

D Pulmonary arterial involvement

E Sparing of brachiocephalic artery

Answer on page 74

QUESTION 88

A 49-year-old man presents to his GP with increasing shortness of breath. A CXR demonstrates a 'white out' of the left hemithorax with displacement of the mediastinum towards the left. What is the most likely explanation?

A Diaphragmatic hernia
B Extensive consolidation
C Lung collapse
D Mesothelioma
E Pleural effusion

Answer on page 74

QUESTION 89

Whilst reporting plain radiographs from a respiratory outpatient clinic, you view a CXR that demonstrates bilateral hypertransradiant hemithoraces. The lung volumes are normal and, unfortunately, there is no clinical history accompanying the request card. Which diagnosis would best explain these findings?

A Acute bronchiolitis
B Asthma
C COPD
D Multiple pulmonary emboli
E Tracheal stenosis

Answer on page 74

QUESTION 90

A CXR is performed on a 62-year-old man with a chronic cough. This demonstrates multiple tiny nodules throughout both lungs, measuring up to 2 mm in size. These micronodules appear to be of greater density than soft tissue. Which one of the following is the most likely diagnosis?

A Coal worker's pneumoconiosis

B Miliary histoplasmosis

C Miliary tuberculosis

D Sarcoidosis

E Silicosis

Answer on page 75

QUESTION 91

A 51-year-old man presents to his GP with hypertension and intermittent headaches. A CXR is performed and demonstrates inferior rib notching. The initial working diagnosis is coarctation of the aorta, but which additional diagnosis should also be considered?

A Marfan's syndrome

B Neurofibromatosis Type I

C Rheumatoid arthritis

D Scleroderma

E Systemic lupus erythematosus

Answer on page 75

QUESTION 92

A 22-year-old man has been involved in a road traffic accident and sustained a comminuted open fracture of his left femur. No other major traumatic injury is identified. Approximately 48 hours later, he becomes acutely short of breath with the development of widespread ill-defined peripheral infiltrates on a supine CXR. His heart size is normal and no pleural effusions are demonstrated. Which one of the following is the most likely diagnosis?

A Cardiogenic pulmonary oedema

B Fat emboli

C Hospital acquired pneumonia

D Löffler's syndrome

E Pulmonary contusions

Answer on page 75

QUESTION 93

A 58-year-old woman presents to her GP with increasing shortness of breath and a dry cough. A CXR demonstrates a reticular interstitial pattern with a 'honeycomb' appearance of multiple cystic spaces in the lower zones. Which one of the following is the most likely diagnosis?

A Extrinsic allergic alveolitis

B Langerhans cell histiocytosis

C Previous radiation therapy

D Rheumatoid lung

E Sarcoidosis

Answer on page 75

QUESTION 94

A 30-year-old man suffers blunt trauma to the right side of the chest after falling off a horse. A contrast-enhanced CT chest and abdomen is performed and demonstrates pulmonary contusions in the right lung. A thin-walled cystic space is noted within the otherwise normal left lung. What is the most likely diagnosis?

A Cystic adenomatoid malformation

B Klippel Trenaunay Weber syndrome

C Lymphangioleiomyomatosis

D Pneumatocoele

E Septic emboli

Answer on page 76

QUESTION 95

A 50-year-old man has entered a drug trial which requires a CXR as part of the protocol. The reporting radiologist has noticed a solitary pulmonary nodule measuring 2 cm in diameter, within the right mid zone. There is no associated pulmonary, pleural or mediastinal lymphadenopathy. Which additional finding is likely to suggest that this is a malignant mass?

A A doubling time of less than 2 weeks

B Enhancement <15 HU post contrast medium administration

C Laminated calcification

D Lobulated margin

E Well-defined margins

Answer on page 76

QUESTION 96

You are asked by the Emergency Department clinicians to review a trauma series of plain radiographs of a young man involved in a road traffic accident. The clinicians suspect that the patient has multiple right-sided rib fractures. Which one of the following is the correct radiological consideration as you review these films?

A A double fracture of a single rib leads to a 'flail segment'.

B Fractures of the 1st to 3rd ribs imply a minor trauma.

C If fractures of the 10th to 12th ribs are present, further imaging is likely to be required.

D Rib fractures are commonly seen in children.

E The supine chest radiograph is a sensitive screening test for rib fractures.

Answer on page 76

QUESTION 97

A 75-year-old man presents to his GP with a persistent cough, green sputum and fevers. A CXR demonstrates basal consolidation with an upwardly concave meniscus, travelling up the lateral chest wall. An ultrasound of the chest demonstrates a hypoechoic pleural collection with internal septations and debris. Pleural aspiration is remarkable for normal pH and protein concentration of 44g/L. What is the most likely cause for this effusion?

A Cardiac failure

B Empyema

C Pancreatitis

D Parapneumonic effusion

E Pulmonary infarction

Answer on page 76

QUESTION 98

A 45-year-old woman presents with pyrexia, cough, weight loss and night sweats of three months' duration. She is found to have a peripheral eosinophilia and a CXR reveals patchy, nonsegmental consolidation in the periphery of the mid and upper zones. The radiographic changes rapidly resolve with corticosteroid therapy. Which one of the following was the most likely diagnosis?

A Chronic eosinophilic pneumonia

B Churg Strauss syndrome

C Invasive aspergillosis

D Simple pulmonary eosinophilia (Löffler's syndrome)

E Tuberculosis

Answer on page 77

QUESTION 99

A 27-year-old woman has severe asthma. She is admitted to ITU with a severe, life-threatening exacerbation requiring mechanical ventilation. Two days later, a supine CXR is performed. This demonstrates a lucent line around the left heart border and aortic arch with surgical emphysema at the root of the neck. The lungs are hyperinflated but appear clear. Which complication is likely to have occurred?

A Alveolar rupture

B Diaphragmatic rupture

C Oesophageal perforation

D Pneumothorax

E Tracheobronchial rupture

Answer on page 77

QUESTION 100

A 57-year-old woman recently underwent palliative chemotherapy for a locally invasive right breast cancer. She now presents with increased cough and breathlessness and a CXR is performed. This demonstrates thickened septal lines with reticulonodular interstitial opacification in the right mid and lower zones. The left lung is clear but a small right pleural effusion is noted. What is the most likely diagnosis?

   A Cryptogenic organising pneumonitis
   B Drug-induced fibrosis
   C Lymphangitis carcinomatosa
   D Pulmonary metastases
   E Pneumocystis jiroveci (PCP)

Answer on page 77

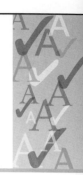

Cardiothoracic and Vascular

ANSWERS

QUESTION 1

ANSWER: C

Sarcoidosis is a disease of young adults commonly presenting with bilateral symmetrical lymphadenopathy; only occasionally appearing in an asymmetrical distribution.

Reference: *Grainger & Allison's* 5e, pp 248, 276, 357, 359, 371.

QUESTION 2

ANSWER: C

Direct and indirect insults to the lung can result in increased permeability of the pulmonary vasculature allowing protein-rich fluid to pass into the alveolar spaces at normal hydrostatic pressures. ARDS is the more severe form of this disease and the earliest radiographic findings are patchy ill-defined airspace opacities in both lungs.

Reference: *Grainger & Allison's* 5e, pp 390–391.

QUESTION 3

ANSWER: C

Allergic bronchopulmonary aspergillosis (ABPA) is part of a spectrum of disease caused by *Aspergillus fumigatus*. Hypersensitive individuals (commonly those with asthma) can present with ABPA and the key radiological features are central airway mucoid impaction leading to central bronchiectasis.

Reference: *Grainger & Allison's* 5e, pp 281 and 301.

QUESTION 4

ANSWER: E

In lung cancer, the radiological pattern of disease varies with the cell type. Squamous cell tumours are the most common tumour to cavitate and those most frequently associated with collapse/consolidation of the lung due to their predominantly central location.

Reference: *Grainger & Allison's* 5e, pp 328–329.

QUESTION 5

ANSWER: D

T3 and T4 tumours can be of any size. However, if the tumour extends into the chest wall, diaphragm or the mediastinal pleura or pericardium (without involving the heart or mediastinal structures) it is a T3 tumour.

Reference: *Grainger & Allison's* 5e, p 331.

QUESTION 6

ANSWER: A

A normal chest radiograph is the most common finding in the setting of a suspected pulmonary embolus (PE).

Reference: *Grainger & Allison's* 5e, pp 537–538.

QUESTION 7

ANSWER: A

Panlobular emphysema is seen in α1-antitrypsin deficiency. The disease tends to occur in a lower lobe distribution (unless there is a smoking history, where an upper lobe predominance can be seen).

Reference: *Grainger & Allison's* 5e, pp 302–304.

QUESTION 8

ANSWER: D

Pulmonary agenesis and hypoplasia is usually asymptomatic with mediastinal displacement towards a dense hemithorax. Poliomyelitis can cause atrophy of the overlying pectoral muscles. MacLeod's syndrome is a late sequel of childhood bronchiolitis with a small lung, small pulmonary arteries and expiratory air trapping on the affected side. If there is an embolus lodged in a major pulmonary artery, the vessels distal to the obstruction will be underperfused with associated loss of lung volume.

Reference: Chapman S, Nakielny R. *Aids to Radiological Differential Diagnosis*, 5th edition (Edinburgh: Saunders, 2003), pp 63–64.

QUESTION 9

ANSWER: A

A transudate is defined as a fluid collection with a low protein concentration (< 30 g/L), whereas an exudate has a high protein concentration (> 30 g/L). Cardiac failure increases the capillary hydrostatic pressure which forces protein poor fluid across intact membranes. Any pathological process that leads to damage of cell membranes will allow the passage of protein macromolecules through the membrane and consequently an exudate.

Reference: Chapman S, Nakielny R. *A Guide to Radiological Procedures*, 4th edition (Edinburgh: Saunders, 2003), pp 93–95.

QUESTION 10

ANSWER: C

Coarctation of the aorta is associated with inferior rib notching (which takes several years to develop) and the resultant hypertension often produces left ventricular hypertrophy. The first two ribs are generally spared as the intercostal arteries are supplied via the costocervical trunk proximal to the coarctation and therefore do not contribute to the collateral circulation.

Reference: *Grainger & Allison's* 5e, p 551.

QUESTION 11

ANSWER: D

Pectus excavatum is often an isolated abnormality but may be associated with Marfan's syndrome or congenital heart disease.

Reference: *Grainger & Allison's* 5e, p 221.

QUESTION 12

ANSWER: B

A number of drugs have been described as causing pleural effusions, the most common agents being cytotoxics (eg bleomycin). Antimigraine agents, amiodarone, bromocriptine and gonadotrophins are also associated with pleural effusions.

Reference: *Grainger & Allison's* 5e, p 227.

QUESTION 13

ANSWER: B

Typical signs of a pneumothorax are seen on the erect radiograph where pleural air rises to the apex. Here the visceral pleural line at the apex becomes separated from the chest wall by a transradiant zone devoid of vessels.

Reference: *Grainger & Allison's* 5e, pp 228–229.

QUESTION 14

ANSWER: B

Hypertrophic osteoarthropathy is a well-recognised complication seen with a localised mesothelioma.

Reference: *Grainger & Allison's* 5e, pp 232–233.

QUESTION 15

ANSWER: A

Bronchogenic cysts are the most common intrathoracic foregut cyst.

Reference: *Grainger & Allison's* 5e, pp 253–254.

QUESTION 16

ANSWER: D

Superior vena cava obstruction is the most common complication of fibrosing mediastinitis, but occasionally it can present with pulmonary arterial obstruction, pulmonary venous obstruction (peribronchial obstruction, septal lines etc), central airway narrowing (stridor) and oesophageal narrowing (dysphagia).

Reference: *Grainger & Allison's* 5e, pp 258–259.

QUESTION 17

ANSWER: B

Lymphangiomas (cystic hygromas) are congenital malformations of the lymphatic system presenting as prevascular masses and comprising complex cystic spaces with the attenuation of the contents close to water on CT.

Reference: *Grainger & Allison's* 5e, pp 256–257.

QUESTION 18

ANSWER: E

Many community-acquired pneumonias are caused by *Streptococcus pneumoniae* with radiographic features of peripheral, homogeneous opacification. Air bronchograms may be present, but cavitation and empyema are uncommon.

Reference: *Grainger & Allison's* 5e, pp 269, 273.

QUESTION 19

ANSWER: A

Klebsiella pneumoniae leads to an extensive exudative response leading to cavitating lobar consolidation and bulging fissures. Legionnaire's disease, on the other hand, tends to present with multifocal lobar, homogeneous opacities with a tendency to appear like masses.

Reference: *Grainger & Allison's* 5e, p 271.

QUESTION 20

ANSWER B

Primary tuberculosis causes a pneumonia that mimics *Streptococcus pneumoniae* in its radiographic appearance and, in children, lymphadenopathy is the most common manifestation.

Reference: *Grainger & Allison's* 5e, pp 276–277.

QUESTION 21

ANSWER: C

Histoplasma capsulatum is a fungus found in moist soil and bird/bat excreta and histoplasmosis occurs most commonly in areas of construction or regions near bat caves. A 'target' lesion describes a solitary, well-defined nodule (a histoplasmoma) with central calcification and is very specific for this condition.

Reference: *Grainger & Allison's* 5e, pp 279–280.

QUESTION 22

ANSWER: C

Hydatid cyst rupture can lead to a variety of appearances: an air–fluid level, a floating membrane (the water lily sign), crumpled membranes in the dependent part of the cyst and a cyst with all contents expectorated (empty cyst sign).

Reference: *Grainger & Allison's* 5e, pp 283–284.

QUESTION 23

ANSWER: E

Pneumatocoeles will generally disappear over time and the majority of radiological signs of PCP will resolve with treatment.

Reference: *Grainger & Allison's* 5e, pp 284–289.

QUESTION 24

ANSWER: B

Mounier-Kuhn disease (tracheobronchomegaly) describes patients with marked dilatation of the trachea and mainstream bronchi and is a radiological diagnosis.

Reference: *Grainger & Allison's* 5e, pp 294–296.

QUESTION 25

ANSWER: E

Bronchiectasis (irreversible dilatation of the bronchi) is classified into three pathological subtypes of increasing severity: cylindrical (relatively uniform airway dilatation), varicose (the bronchial lumen assumes a beaded configuration) and cystic (a string or cluster of cystic structures).

Reference: *Grainger & Allison's* 5e, pp 297–299.

QUESTION 26

ANSWER: C

Recurrent, long courses of intravenous antibiotics often lead to medium/long-term venous access in patients with CF. Bronchiectasis is seen in a predominantly upper lobe distribution, with mucus plugging and hyperinflation.

Reference: *Grainger & Allison's* 5e, p 300.

QUESTION 27

ANSWER: D

Obliterative bronchiolitis describes bronchiolar and peribronchiolar inflammation affecting the membranous and respiratory bronchioles. Affected areas display decreased attenuation as a result of air trapping and decreased perfusion relative to normal areas.

Reference: *Grainger & Allison's* 5e, pp 308, 409.

QUESTION 28

ANSWER: C

The collapsed right middle lobe will lie adjacent to the right heart border and as there is no longer a clear heart–lung interface, then the right heart border appears indistinct.

Reference: *Grainger & Allison's* 5e, p 320.

QUESTION 29

ANSWER: B

Left upper lobe collapse results in volume loss in an anterior and medial direction, as opposed to superior and medial collapse of the right upper lobe collapse.

Reference: *Grainger & Allison's* 5e, pp 318–320.

QUESTION 30

ANSWER: E

Squamous cell carcinoma of the lung is the most common bronchogenic carcinoma to demonstrate cavitation.

Reference: *Grainger & Allison's* 5e, pp 281, 329, 535.

QUESTION 31

ANSWER: A

Most bronchial carcinoids arise in the central airways and are often seen with collapse/consolidation of distal lung, due to bronchial obstruction.

Reference: *Grainger & Allison's* 5e, p 338.

QUESTION 32

ANSWER: A

At presentation, Hodgkin's disease most commonly has lung parenchymal disease accompanied by intrathoracic adenopathy, whereas isolated lung involvement is not uncommon in non-Hodgkin's lymphoma. Pleural effusions (unilateral) are common in both types of lymphoma, as are peripheral subpleural masses. Consolidation with air bronchograms can also be seen in both diseases.

Reference: *Grainger & Allison's* 5e, pp 340, 1740–1741.

QUESTION 33

ANSWER: C

Calcified lung metastases rarely occur, except in osteosarcoma and chondrosarcoma. Even if a primary tumour displays calcification (eg breast or colonic carcinoma), the pulmonary metastases will rarely demonstrate calcification.

Reference: *Grainger & Allison's* 5e, p 342.

QUESTION 34

ANSWER: E

The above HRCT findings are almost pathognomonic for UIP and when a confident diagnosis of UIP is made on HRCT it is usually correct.

Reference: *Grainger & Allison's* 5e, pp 352–354.

QUESTION 35

ANSWER: D

NSIP is characterised by interstitial inflammation and fibrosis, but without any of the specific features that allow a diagnosis of UIP to be made. NSIP is usually of uniform temporality and has a more prominent ground glass component than the reticular pattern seen in UIP.

Reference: *Grainger & Allison's* 5e, pp 352–354.

QUESTION 36

ANSWER: C

Sarcoidosis has traditionally been staged according to chest radiograph appearances: Stage 0—normal chest radiograph, Stage I—bilateral hilar adenopathy, Stage II—bilateral hilar adenopathy and parenchymal involvement, Stage III—parenchymal involvement with shrinking adenopathy, Stage IV—parenchymal volume loss as a result of pulmonary fibrosis.

Reference: *Grainger & Allison's* 5e, p 357.

QUESTION 37

ANSWER: D

Reference: *Grainger & Allison's* 5e, pp 352, 358, 360–362.

QUESTION 38

ANSWER: D

Extrinsic allergic alveolitis is an immunologically mediated lung disease as a result of exposure to lung antigens, including those found in paint sprays.

Reference: *Grainger & Allison's* 5e, pp 355, 359.

QUESTION 39

ANSWER: A

LCH is most commonly seen in men (4:1) and the vast majority of patients are cigarette smokers (the converse is true for lymphangioleiomyomatosis).

Reference: *Grainger & Allison's* 5e, pp 361–362.

QUESTION 40

ANSWER: C

Rheumatoid arthritis is associated with pleural effusions/thickening, interstitial fibrosis, bronchiectasis and bronchiolitis. Necrobiotic nodules are uncommon and are usually associated with subcutaneous nodules.

Reference: *Grainger & Allison's* 5e, pp 362–363.

QUESTION 41

ANSWER: E

Pleuro-pulmonary disease is very common in SLE, occurring in over 50% of patients at some stage during the course of their disease. This often manifests as relatively small bilateral pleural effusions, associated with pleuritic chest pain.

Reference: *Grainger & Allison's* 5e, p 365.

QUESTION 42

ANSWER: C

Wegener's granulomatosis is characterised by necrotising granulomatous inflammation of the upper and lower respiratory tracts and is associated with glomerulonephritis. The most common radiological finding is cavitating lung masses measuring up to 10 cm in diameter.

Reference: *Grainger & Allison's* 5e, p 366.

QUESTION 43

ANSWER: D

Silicosis and CWP both result in small, well-defined nodules with an upper lobe distribution. As the nodules enlarge they can coalesce and form mass-like opacities with upper lobe contraction (progressive massive fibrosis). This is much more commonly seen in silicosis.

Reference: *Grainger & Allison's* 5e, pp 371–372.

QUESTION 44

ANSWER: B

Asbestos-related pleural plaques involve the parietal pleura almost exclusively and the classic locations are along the posterolateral and lateral chest walls, the diaphragmatic dome and mediastinal pleura. Calcified diaphragmatic plaques are virtually pathognomonic of asbestos exposure.

Reference: *Grainger & Allison's* 5e, p 372.

QUESTION 45

ANSWER: B

Round atelectasis (folded lung) is a benign condition seen in patients exposed to asbestos.

Reference: *Grainger & Allison's* 5e, p 372.

QUESTION 46

ANSWER: B

Fractures of the 1st to 3rd ribs imply severe trauma and can be associated with vascular, neural, spinal or tracheobronchial injuries.

Reference: *Grainger & Allison's* 5e, p 380.

QUESTION 47

ANSWER: B

Known as the 'deep sulcus sign'. A visible pleural line due to a pneumothorax is more commonly seen on an erect rather than supine CXR.

Reference: *Grainger & Allison's* 5e, p 381.

QUESTION 48

ANSWER: E

Abdominal contents passing into the right hemithorax via a right diaphragmatic rupture will push the mediastinal structures towards the left. Hollow viscera within the chest are more commonly seen in a left diaphragmatic rupture as the liver will tend to obstruct the passage of abdominal contents into the chest (the same will apply for a nasogastric tube).

Reference: *Grainger & Allison's* 5e, p 384.

QUESTION 49

ANSWER: E

The target sign is seen in intussusception and consists of two concentric circles of fat density alternating with soft tissue density. The other signs can all be seen in diaphragmatic rupture.

Reference: *Grainger & Allison's* 5e, pp 384, 595.

QUESTION 50

ANSWER: D

Tracheobronchial rupture is rare and occurs when significant compressive force is applied to the chest. It is associated with upper rib, thoracic spine and sternal fractures and, if a mainstem bronchus is completely ruptured, the remaining intact vessels cannot support the lung hilum, resulting in the lung 'falling' within the hemithorax (the 'fallen lung' sign).

Reference: *Grainger & Allison's* 5e, p 386.

QUESTION 51

ANSWER: A

Signs of a mediastinal haematoma (and possible aortic rupture) include widening of the mediastinum (greater than 8 cm above the level of the carina or more than 25% of the width of the chest at this level), a left apical pleural cap or pleural effusion and deviation of the trachea to the right.

Reference: *Grainger & Allison's* 5e, p 387.

QUESTION 52

ANSWER: E

ARDS results from insults to the lung either from direct (eg pneumonia) or indirect (eg pancreatitis) causes and develops through three phases: exudative, proliferative and finally fibrotic.

Reference: *Grainger & Allison's* 5e, pp 390–391.

QUESTION 53

ANSWER: D

Aspiration is predisposed in patients with a reduced consciousness level and pulmonary changes tend to occur within hours following aspiration and regress 72 hours later.

Reference: *Grainger & Allison's* 5e, p 389.

QUESTION 54

ANSWER: B

The most common causes of pulmonary oedema in the ITU patient are cardiac failure and overhydration and may be radiologically indistinguishable. Overhydration will tend to cause a more central distribution of oedema and a wider vascular pedicle.

Reference: *Grainger & Allison's* 5e, p 389.

QUESTION 55

ANSWER: E

The tip of an endotracheal tube should lie at least 5 cm above the carina, allowing a degree of upward and downward movement (as a result of head motion) and avoiding inadvertent intubation of the right main bronchus. Central venous pressure catheters and peripherally inserted central catheter lines should lie within the superior vena cava. A nasogastric tube should lie in the left upper quadrant of the abdomen with the side holes seen within the stomach.

Reference: *Grainger & Allison's* 5e, pp 392–393.

QUESTION 56

ANSWER: A

Acute rejection has nonspecific radiological findings with persisting airspace opacities developing at day 5–10 postoperatively.

Reference: *Grainger & Allison's* 5e, pp 393–394.

QUESTION 57

ANSWER: A

Comparing the air density in an airway with the lung parenchyma (the 'black bronchus' sign) can help with the detection of subtle ground glass change (the two densities are usually equivalent).

Reference: *Grainger & Allison's* 5e, pp 403–404.

QUESTION 58

ANSWER: A

Idiopathic pulmonary fibrosis presents with peripheral reticular opacities predominantly at the lung bases within which there are areas of honeycomb destruction.

Reference: *Grainger & Allison's* 5e, pp 352, 404–406.

QUESTION 59

ANSWER: E

Pulmonary oedema results from the passage of fluid from the intravascular space to the alveoli, initially via the interstitium. Oedema of the perivascular interstitium can lead to thickening of the airway walls and peribronchial cuffing.

Reference: *Grainger & Allison's* 5e, pp 405–407.

QUESTION 60

ANSWER: E

Wegener's granulomatosis is a multisystem disease, commonly affecting the respiratory and renal tracts. In most patients there are multiple nodules which can cavitate and infarct, leading to surrounding areas of ground glass attenuation.

Reference: *Grainger & Allison's* 5e, p 409.

QUESTION 61

ANSWER: A

The radiographic changes of alveolar proteinosis are mostly nonspecific with airspace opacification in a predominantly central location. HRCT features are more specific for alveolar proteinosis with a 'crazy paving' pattern due to geographical ground glass opacification and thickened interlobular septa.

Reference: *Grainger & Allison's* 5e, p 414.

QUESTION 62

ANSWER: E

Cardiomegaly is a useful sign in detecting structural heart disease. It is most commonly the result of ventricular enlargement, whereas atrial enlargement and pericardial effusion are far less common causes.

Reference: *Grainger & Allison's* 5e, pp 263, 467, 496.

QUESTION 63

ANSWER: E

Constrictive pericarditis is usually associated with obliteration of the pericardial cavity, so radiological signs of a pericardial effusion (effacement of the heart borders, bilateral hilar overlay, filling in of the retrosternal space and the epicardial fat pad sign) will tend to be absent.

Reference: *Grainger & Allison's* 5e, p 263.

QUESTION 64

ANSWER: D

The cardinal feature of rheumatic mitral valve disease is left atrial enlargement (particularly affecting the left atrial appendage in rheumatic disease). Enlargement of the left ventricle is not a feature of mitral stenosis but can be seen with severe mitral regurgitation.

Reference: *Grainger & Allison's* 5e, pp 470–472.

QUESTION 65

ANSWER: D

Carcinoid syndrome can cause subendocardial fibroelastosis with thickening and shortening of the tricuspid valve cusps. This usually leads to tricuspid regurgitation but can sometime cause tricuspid stenosis.

Reference: *Grainger & Allison's* 5e, p 474.

QUESTION 66

ANSWER: C

The clinical features of rheumatic aortic stenosis are similar to calcific aortic stenosis but with a few caveats. Rheumatic aortic disease is commonly associated with rheumatic mitral disease leading to left atrial enlargement and significant dyspnoea.

Reference: *Grainger & Allison's* 5e, pp 476–477.

QUESTION 67

ANSWER: E

Hypertrophic cardiomyopathy is characterised by marked hypertrophy of the left ventricular myocardium with good or even hyperdynamic contractility. Altered flow dynamics can cause the mitral valve to be compressed against the interventricular septum, partially obstructing the subaortic region—known as systolic anterior motion of the mitral valve.

Reference: *Grainger & Allison's* 5e, pp 488–492.

QUESTION 68

ANSWER: C

Primary cardiac tumours are rare and occur less frequently than metastatic tumours to the heart. If a primary cardiac tumour has a narrow attachment to the cardiac wall, then it is more likely to be a benign lesion than a malignant primary cardiac tumour.

Reference: *Grainger & Allison's* 5e, p 495.

QUESTION 69

ANSWER: D

Cardiac myxoma is the most common cardiac tumour with 75% occurring within the left atrium.

Reference: *Grainger & Allison's* 5e, pp 496–500.

QUESTION 70

ANSWER: E

Myocardial ischaemia is associated with reduced cardiac contractility and therefore reduced wall motion on cardiac MR and echocardiography. Reduced distortion of the tagging grid on cardiac MR occurs due to the reduced wall motion.

Reference: *Grainger & Allison's* 5e, pp 506–510.

QUESTION 71

ANSWER: A

In the few days following myocardial infarction there may be high myocardial signal seen on T2w images. A recent infarct will demonstrate reduced myocardial perfusion with first pass contrast medium imaging but delayed enhancement is seen.

Reference: *Grainger & Allison's* 5e, p 514.

QUESTION 72

ANSWER: C

The normal coronary arterial lumen is initially preserved with atherosclerosis with increasing wall thickness accompanied by an increasing outer vessel wall diameter. Calcification of the coronary arteries is proportional to the degree of coronary arterial stenosis present.

Reference: *Grainger & Allison's* 5e, pp 518–520.

QUESTION 73

ANSWER: A

PVH occurs as a result of increased resistance in the pulmonary veins most commonly as a result of left-sided heart disease.

Reference: *Grainger & Allison's* 5e, p 532.

QUESTION 74

ANSWER: E

Certain patterns of opacification may suggest a certain diagnosis. Severe mitral regurgitation is associated with opacification within the right upper zone resulting from regurgitant blood flow in the right upper lobe pulmonary artery from the superoposteriorly positioned mitral valve.

Reference: *Grainger & Allison's* 5e, pp 390, 531.

QUESTION 75

ANSWER: B

Chronic pulmonary arterial hypertension is characterised by enlargement of the central pulmonary arteries (with a diameter greater than that of the adjacent ascending aorta) with associated tapering of the peripheral arterial branches at the segmental level (peripheral pruning).

Reference: *Grainger & Allison's* 5e, p 532.

QUESTION 76

ANSWER: A

MacLeod's syndrome (Swyer James syndrome) is a manifestation of childhood postinfectious obliterative bronchiolitis, resulting in diminished vascularity and reduced growth of the affected lung.

Reference: *Grainger & Allison's* 5e, p 534.

QUESTION 77

ANSWER: A

Reference: *Grainger & Allison's* 5e, pp 277, 533, 534.

QUESTION 78

ANSWER: A

In the acute setting enlargement of the central pulmonary arteries is rare—this is more commonly seen with chronic repeated embolic disease and the subsequent development of pulmonary arterial hypertension.

Reference: *Grainger & Allison's* 5e, p 538.

QUESTION 79

ANSWER: E

In patients with COPD, pleural effusions, consolidation and lobar collapse pulmonary hypoxic vasoconstriction reduces blood flow to poorly ventilated areas of lung. If this process is not complete a 'reversed mismatch' can occur where there is more prominent ventilation than perfusion.

Reference: *Grainger & Allison's* 5e, p 538.

QUESTION 80

ANSWER: E

On CTPA, an acute PE is seen as an intravascular filling defect. If contrast medium flows around the thrombus, then a 'tram track' appearance can be seen.

Reference: *Grainger & Allison's* 5e, p 540.

QUESTION 81

ANSWER: B

The most common adult pulmonary metastases arise from breast, kidney, head and neck and gastrointestinal tract tumours.

Reference: *Grainger & Allison's* 5e, pp 342–343.

QUESTION 82

ANSWER: B

On CT peripheral and/or central bronchiectasis is present in all advanced cases of cystic fibrosis.

Reference: *Grainger & Allison's* 5e, p 300.

QUESTION 83

ANSWER: C

Pneumocystis pneumonia typically demonstrates bilateral, symmetrical, fine to medium reticular opacities as opposed to the coarse, reticulonodular pattern seen in patients with advanced HIV and tuberculosis.

Reference: *Grainger & Allison's* 5e, pp 284–286.

QUESTION 84

ANSWER: A

Pleural effusions, cavitation and empyema formation are common with staphylococcal infection, whereas air bronchograms are unusual.

Reference: *Grainger & Allison's* 5e, pp 269–273.

QUESTION 85

ANSWER: E

'Foregut duplication cysts' describe those congenital cysts derived from the embryological foregut and includes bronchogenic, enteric and neurenteric cysts. Neurenteric cysts are found in the posterior mediastinum (with associated vertebral anomalies) and frequently produce pain.

Reference: *Grainger & Allison's* 5e, pp 252–253.

QUESTION 86

ANSWER: C

Aortic dissections affecting the descending aorta only (origin distal to the left subclavian artery) are classified as DeBakey type III dissection (Stanford type B). A type IIIa dissection is limited to the thoracic aorta, whereas if there is extension involving the abdominal aorta, it is classified as DeBakey type IIIb dissection.

Reference: *Grainger & Allison's* 5e, p 557.

QUESTION 87

ANSWER: D

Granulomatous vasculitis (Takayasu's disease) is a chronic inflammatory disease involving the aorta (and its main branches) and pulmonary arteries leading to stenosis, occlusion or dilatation.

Reference: *Grainger & Allison's* 5e, pp 562–563.

QUESTION 88

ANSWER: C

Increased density of a hemithorax with a central mediastinum can be seen with consolidation, mesothelioma and pleural effusions. If an effusion is large enough the hemithorax is likely to be displaced away from the abnormal hemithorax (this is also seen with a diaphragmatic hernia). Causes of a dense hemithorax and mediastinal shift towards the affected side include collapse, post pneumonectomy, lymphangitis carcinomatosis and pulmonary agenesis / hypoplasia.

Reference: Chapman & Nakielny, *Aids to Radiological Differential Diagnosis*, p 66.

QUESTION 89

ANSWER: D

Multiple pulmonary emboli can lead to pulmonary arterial pruning and increased transradiancy in normal volume lungs. The overinflation seen in asthma is secondary to bronchial constriction and mucus plugging, whereas bronchial inflammation can lead to overinflation seen in bronchiolitis. Tracheal stenosis will also impair the expiratory phase of ventilation, also potentially leading to overinflation.

Reference: Chapman & Nakielny, *Aids to Radiological Differential Diagnosis*, pp 63–64.

QUESTION 90

ANSWER: E

Silicosis often demonstrates multiple well-defined nodules, which can appear very dense due to the pure silica deposits. The other conditions listed here can also demonstrate multiple opacities of varying morphology, but these are typically of soft tissue density.

Reference: Chapman & Nakielny, *Aids to Radiological Differential Diagnosis*, pp 481–482.

QUESTION 91

ANSWER: B

Neurofibromatosis type 1 is a well-recognised cause of inferior rib notching.

Reference: *Grainger & Allison's* 5e, pp 220–221.

QUESTION 92

ANSWER: B

Fat emboli typically present 1–2 days post trauma and resolve in 1–4 weeks. As it is an embolic phenomenon, neurological and skin abnormalities can occur. The normal heart size and absence of effusions make cardiogenic oedema unlikely.

References: Chapman & Nakielny, *Aids to Radiological Differential Diagnosis*, p 88. *Grainger & Allison's* 5e, p 412.

QUESTION 93

ANSWER: D

Rheumatoid fibrosis demonstrates predominantly basal changes, whilst the other conditions listed here typically produce interstitial changes in different distributions.

References: Chapman & Nakielny, *Aids to Radiological Differential Diagnosis*, pp 77–78, 472. *Grainger & Allison's* 5e, pp 300, 358.

QUESTION 94

ANSWER: D

Severe blunt trauma may introduce shearing forces within the lung and, if the resultant tear fills with air, a pneumatocoele can form. Cystic adenomatoid malformations usually present in early childhood, whilst lymphangioleiomyomatosis is only seen in females.

References: Chapman & Nakielny, *Aids to Radiological Differential Diagnosis*, p 87. *Grainger & Allison's* 5e, p 382.

QUESTION 95

ANSWER: D

The most important criteria distinguishing benign from malignant solitary pulmonary nodules are the nodule attenuation and growth over time. Lobulation of a mass suggests uneven growth rates in a tumour mass.

Reference: *Grainger & Allison's* 5e, pp 326, 344–346.

QUESTION 96

ANSWER: C

As fractures of the 10th to 12th ribs are frequently associated with liver, splenic and renal injuries, further imaging is usually required.

Reference: *Grainger & Allison's* 5e, pp 379–380.

QUESTION 97

ANSWER: D

The ultrasound and pleural fluid features are those of an exudative pleural effusion. The normal pH makes an empyema unlikely and a parapneumonic effusion is the most likely diagnosis.

Reference: Chapman & Nakielny, *A Guide to Radiological Procedures*, 4th edition (Edinburgh: Saunders, 2003), pp 93–95.

QUESTION 98

ANSWER: A

Patients with simple pulmonary eosinophilia typically have a self-limiting mild respiratory illness with a peripheral eosinophilia. Chronic eosinophilic pneumonia is associated with a more severe and prolonged illness with characteristic mid and upper zone peripheral infiltrates ('reverse bats wing' appearance) that resolve rapidly with corticosteroids.

Reference: *Grainger & Allison's* 5e, pp 412–413.

QUESTION 99

ANSWER: A

The clinical and radiographic appearances are those of a pneumomediastinum. Asthma and mechanical ventilation are risk factors for alveolar rupture, with gas tracking back through the peribronchovascular sheath to the mediastinum.

Reference: *Grainger & Allison's* 5e, pp 385–386.

QUESTION 100

ANSWER: C

The most common causes of lymphangitis carcinomatosa are lung and breast cancer.

Reference: *Grainger & Allison's* 5e, pp 343–344.

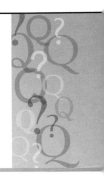

MODULE 2

Musculoskeletal and Trauma

QUESTIONS

QUESTION 1

An athletic 19-year-old medical student presents to the Emergency Department after sustaining an injury to his right hip during training. A radiograph reveals a fracture of the anterior superior iliac spine. What is the most likely diagnosis?

A Avulsion of the adductor muscles

B Avulsion of the hamstring muscles

C Avulsion of iliopsoas

D Avulsion of rectus femoris

E Avulsion of sartorius

Answer on page 120

QUESTION 2

The radiograph of an 8-year-old boy with dietary Vitamin D deficiency reveals cupping and fraying of the distal tibial metaphysis. Which radiological finding is a recognised feature of this condition?

A Cortical sclerosis involving the margin of the epiphysis

B Expansion of the costochondral junctions

C Exuberant periosteal reaction

D Increased density of the end of the metaphyses

E Metaphyseal spurs

Answer on page 120

QUESTION 3

A 60-year-old woman is assessed by the Emergency Department following a fall onto her right wrist. The initial radiograph shows an extra-articular fracture of the right distal radius, with volar subluxation of the distal fragment. Which eponymous fracture type best matches this description?

A Barton's fracture

B Colles' fracture

C Hutchinson's fracture

D Reverse Barton's fracture

E Smith's fracture

Answer on page 121

QUESTION 4

A previously well 80-year-old woman sustains a subcapital fracture of the right neck of femur following a fall onto hard ground. The plain film reveals multiple lytic lesions within the pelvic bones and proximal femora, which are highly suspicious for bone metastases. What is the most likely occult primary lesion?

A Carcinoma of the bladder
B Carcinoma of the breast
C Carcinoma of the bronchus
D Carcinoma of the colon
E Carcinoma of the stomach

Answer on page 121

QUESTION 5

A 32-year-old builder is brought to the Emergency Department following a fall from scaffolding. He is believed to have fallen a considerable height and witnesses report that he landed on his feet. On primary survey, he is tachycardic, hypotensive and extremely tender on palpation of the pelvis and left hip. During resuscitation, a radiographic trauma series is obtained. What is the most likely pattern of pelvic injury?

A Bilateral fractures of the superior and inferior pubic rami
B Bilateral fractures of the superior and inferior pubic rami with a fracture through the left sacral ala
C Disruption of the sacroiliac joints and pubic symphysis
D Localised fracture through the left iliac wing
E Vertical fracture through the left ilium with fractures through the left superior and inferior pubic rami

Answer on page 121

QUESTION 6

A 43-year-old man is investigated for pain related to his left arm. Plain radiography demonstrates a well-defined, lytic lesion in the proximal humerus, with chondroid matrix mineralisation and a narrow zone of transition. There is deep endosteal cortical scalloping and the suggestion of bone expansion. What is the most likely diagnosis?

A Chondroblastoma

B Chondroma

C Chondromyxofibroma

D Chondrosarcoma

E Osteochondroma

Answer on page 121

QUESTION 7

A 19-year-old man, the unrestrained driver in a high-energy road traffic accident, has been brought by ambulance to the Emergency Department. A lateral cervical spine radiograph shows an anterior wedge fracture of C5 with a retropulsed bony fragment. What was the likely predominant force acting on the cervical spine at the time of injury?

A Compression

B Distraction

C Extension

D Flexion

E Shearing

Answer on page 121

QUESTION 8

A 45-year-old man underwent chemotherapy and limb-sparing surgery to treat a soft tissue sarcoma in his left leg. He remains under regular MRI surveillance to detect signs of recurrent disease. What features on MRI would be most suggestive of disease recurrence?

A New areas of high signal on proton density images
B New areas of high signal on T1w images
C New areas of high signal on T2w images
D New areas of reduced signal on T1w images
E New areas of reduced signal on T2w images

Answer on page 121

QUESTION 9

An aggressive, lytic bone lesion is observed to destroy the cortex of the second metacarpal in a 70-year-old woman. What is the most likely cause for these appearances?

A Metastatic breast cancer
B Metastatic colon cancer
C Metastatic lung cancer
D Metastatic renal cancer
E Metastatic thyroid cancer

Answer on page 122

QUESTION 10

A 14-year-old boy attends the Emergency Department following an injury to his right ankle in a rugby match. The radiograph shows a triplane fracture. Which fracture is likely to form part of this complex injury?

A Coronal fracture through the physis

B Coronal fracture through the epiphysis

C Horizontal fracture through the metaphysis.

D Sagittal fracture through the epiphysis

E Sagittal fracture through the metaphysis

Answer on page 122

QUESTION 11

A solitary, lytic lesion with aggressive features is an unexpected incidental finding on radiography of the left knee. Which radiological feature would favour a diagnosis of metastasis rather than primary bone tumour?

A Bone expansion

B Diaphyseal location

C Florid periosteal reaction

D Tumour bone formation

E Soft tissue mass

Answer on page 122

QUESTION 12

A pelvic radiograph reveals a symmetrical abnormality of the proximal femora characterised by thin lucent lines perpendicular to the medial femoral cortex, with a faint sclerotic margin. These linear lucent areas do not extend across the full width of the femur, and the visualised bones are otherwise of normal appearance. Which is the most likely diagnosis?

A Hyperparathyroidism

B Multiple myeloma

C Osteomalacia

D Osteoporosis

E Paget's disease

Answer on page 122

QUESTION 13

A 32-year-old man attends hospital following a fall onto his flexed left arm. He is referred to the duty orthopaedic team with a 'Monteggia injury'. What are the most likely radiological findings?

A A fracture of the distal radius with an associated dislocation of the radial head

B A fracture of the distal radius with an associated disruption of the distal radioulnar joint

C A fracture of the distal ulna with an associated dislocation of the radial head

D A fracture of the proximal ulna with an associated dislocation of the radial head

E A fracture of the proximal radius with an associated disruption of the distal radioulnar joint

Answer on page 123

QUESTION 14

A 1-year-old child with multiple injuries is brought to the Emergency Department by his mother. The history and mechanism of his injuries is not clear. Which radiological finding would be highly specific for non-accidental injury?

A Scapular fracture

B Greenstick fracture

C Linear parietal fracture

D Mid-clavicular fracture

E Single diaphyseal fracture

Answer on page 123

QUESTION 15

A 70-year-old man complains of a tense painless swelling posterior to his right knee. Ultrasound demonstrates a large cyst, which communicates with the knee joint between which two structures?

A Through the interval between semimembranosus and the lateral head of gastrocnemius

B Through the interval between semimembranosus and the medial head of gastrocnemius

C Through the interval between semimembranosus and semitendinosus

D Through the interval between semitendinosus and the lateral head of gastrocnemius

E Through the interval between semitendinosus and the medial head of gastrocnemius

Answer on page 123

QUESTION 16

On an otherwise normal lateral radiograph of the knee, the patella is noted to be inferiorly situated, in keeping with patella baja. What is a possible association of this condition?

 A Cerebral palsy
 B Chondromalacia patella
 C Juvenile idiopathic arthritis
 D Quadriceps atrophy
 E Recurrent patellar subluxation

Answer on page 123

QUESTION 17

A 75-year-old lady undergoes bone mineral density (BMD) measurements at the hip and spine by means of dual energy radiograph absorptiometry (DXA). What findings would satisfy the World Health Organisation (WHO) criteria for osteoporosis?

 A BMD below the young adult reference mean
 B BMD between -1 and -2.5 standard deviations below that of the young adult reference mean
 C BMD more than -2.5 standard deviations below the young adult reference mean
 D BMD more than -2.5 standard deviations below the young adult reference mean, with one low-energy fracture
 E BMD more than -2.5 standard deviations below the young adult reference mean, with two low-energy fractures

Answer on page 123

QUESTION 18

A 27-year-old man is referred by his GP with progressively painful swelling of his left knee following a minor football injury some weeks ago. The radiograph shows a 5-cm ill-defined lytic lesion within the left distal femoral metaphysis, with a permeative pattern of bone loss and areas of cloud-like ossification. There is an extensive periosteal reaction, predominantly orientated perpendicular to the cortex. What is the most likely diagnosis?

A Aneurysmal bone cyst

B Chondrosarcoma

C Ewing's sarcoma

D Metastasis

E Osteosarcoma

Answer on page 123

QUESTION 19

A 25-year-old doctor injures her left wrist whilst snowboarding. Initial radiographs are reported as showing no fracture, but there is clinical suspicion of a scapholunate ligament disruption. Further views are obtained. Which radiological feature would support the diagnosis?

A Scapholunate angle less than 30°

B Scapholunate distance of 2 mm

C 'Signet ring' appearance of the scaphoid

D Rotatory subluxation of the lunate

E Wedge-shaped appearance of the lunate

Answer on page 124

QUESTION 20

A 50-year-old patient with right wrist pain and clicking is referred for a MRI by the orthopaedic surgeons, who suspect ulnolunate impingement. Which of the following imaging features would count against this provisional diagnosis?

A Disruption of the lunotriquetral ligament

B High signal within the lunate on T2w or STIR sequences

C Negative ulnar variance

D Perforation of the central portion of the triangular fibrocartilage (TFC)

E Sclerosis within the lunate

Answer on page 124

QUESTION 21

A 50-year-old woman attends the Emergency Department following a minor hand injury. A plain radiograph reveals no fracture, but there is evidence of subperiosteal erosion along the radial aspect of the middle phalanges of the middle and index fingers. What is the most likely diagnosis?

A Gout

B Hyperparathyroidism

C Myeloma

D Sarcoid

E Systemic lupus erythematosus

Answer on page 124

QUESTION 22

A 6-week-old boy has a positive family history of developmental dysplasia of the hip (DDH) and is referred for a hip ultrasound. Which imaging features would be consistent with normal (Graf type 1) hips?

A Alpha angle greater than 60°

B Beta angle greater than 77°

C Compressed cartilage roof

D Deficient bony roof

E Rounded ossific rim

Answer on page 124

QUESTION 23

An 80-year-old woman is admitted to hospital following a fall. The patient had a right mastectomy and axillary dissection 5 years ago to treat an invasive ductal carcinoma. The pelvic radiograph reveals a left hip fracture. Which fracture site would be most suggestive of a pathological fracture?

A Greater trochanter fracture

B Intertrochanteric fracture of the left proximal femur

C Pertrochanteric fracture of the left proximal femur

D Subcapital fracture of the left neck of femur

E Subtrochanteric fracture of the left proximal femur

Answer on page 124

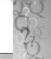

QUESTION 24

Regarding MRI examination of the shoulder, what are the signal characteristics of the normal supraspinatus tendon?

A High signal intensity on all sequences

B High signal on T1w, low signal on T2w

C Intermediate signal on all sequences

D Low signal on all sequences

E Low signal on T1w, high signal on T2w

Answer on page 124

QUESTION 25

A 28-year-old tennis player undergoes a MR arthrogram to investigate recurrent right shoulder instability following a previous glenohumeral dislocation. The MRI reveals a tear of the anterosuperior labrum, closely related to the insertion of the biceps tendon. How are these appearances best described?

A Anterior labral tear

B Bankart lesion

C Hill-Sachs lesion

D Reverse Hill-Sachs lesion

E Superior labrum from anterior to posterior (SLAP) lesion

Answer on page 125

QUESTION 26

In a 40-year-old woman complaining of wrist pain, radiographs reveal sclerosis and collapse of the lunate, with rotatory subluxation of the scaphoid. What is the most likely diagnosis?

A Freiberg's disease

B Kienboeck's disease

C Köhler's disease

D Sever's disease

E Sinding-Larsen disease

Answer on page 125

QUESTION 27

A 30-year-old women experiences, amongst other symptoms, recurrent episodes of painful swelling and stiffness of both hands. Antibodies against antinuclear antigens and double-stranded DNA are detected in peripheral blood samples. Radiographs of both hands are obtained during her assessment. Which radiographic findings are most likely?

A Atrophic soft tissues, resorption of the terminal phalanges and soft tissue calcinosis

B Punched-out marginal erosions in an asymmetric distribution, with preservation of bone density

C Symmetrical abnormality of the MCPs of the index and middle finger, characterised by joint space narrowing, subarticular cysts and hook-like osteophytes

D Symmetrical soft tissue swelling, marginal erosions and juxta-articular osteopaenia

E Ulnar deviation at the MCPJs, without evidence of erosions

Answer on page 125

QUESTION 28

An elderly diabetic patient with an established peripheral sensory neuropathy has deep ulcers on his right foot. Plain films show destruction of the architecture of the midfoot with extensive sclerosis, consistent with a Charcot arthropathy. Which imaging feature would suggest coexistent infection?

A Collapse of the plantar arch on the lateral radiograph

B Enhancement of T1w signal following administration of gadolinium

C Evidence of bone oedema on fluid sensitive sequences

D Reduced bone marrow signal on STIR

E Slow progression of bone destruction on serial radiographs

Answer on page 125

QUESTION 29

A 15-year-old male haemophiliac patient presents to the Emergency Department with painful swelling of the right knee. There have been similar presentations in the past. Following radiographs, he is referred for an MRI of the right knee. Which of the following imaging features would be regarded as unusual or atypical given the history?

A Accelerated maturation of the epiphysis

B Epiphyseal enlargement

C Irregular synovial thickening

D Juxta-articular sclerosis

E Blooming of the synovium on gradient echo sequences

Answer on page 125

QUESTION 30

An asymptomatic 65-year-old woman on long-term steroids for rheumatoid disease undergoes dual energy X-ray absorptiometry (DXA). Her Z score is −2 and her T score is −2.7. What is the WHO definition of osteoporosis?

A T score less than −1
B T score less than −2.5
C Z score less than −1
D Z score less than −2.5
E Mean of T and Z score less than −2

Answer on page 126

QUESTION 31

A 20-year-old footballer injured his ankle 3 months ago, but still experiences pain that prevents a return to competitive sport. An MRI of his injured ankle shows a partially detached osteochondral fragment within the lateral aspect of the talar dome, with fluid deep to the fragment and a fissure in the overlying cartilage. Which stage of disease do these appearances represent?

A Stage 0
B Stage 1
C Stage 2
D Stage 3
E Stage 4

Answer on page 126

QUESTION 32

A young man with sickle cell disease presents to the Emergency Department with left hip pain. The orthopaedic team suspect avascular necrosis and request an MRI of both hips. The MRI shows a subchondral fracture of the left femoral head, with preservation of the joint space. The asymptomatic right hip is normal. How would the appearances of the left hip be classified?

A Stage 0 disease

B Stage I disease

C Stage II disease

D Stage III disease

E Stage IV disease

Answer on page 126

QUESTION 33

A 13-year-old boy is referred to the orthopaedic surgeons with a short history of pain and swelling around his left elbow. The radiograph reveals a 4-cm area of permeative bone destruction within the distal diaphysis of the left humerus, with a wide zone of transition. There is an extensive associated soft tissue component and evidence of a 'hair-on-end' pattern of periosteal reaction. What is most likely diagnosis?

A Askin tumour

B Chondroblastoma

C Chondromyxoid fibroma

D Ewing's sarcoma

E Malignant fibrous histiocytoma

Answer on page 126

QUESTION 34

A 2-cm, well-defined lytic bone lesion in the proximal tibial metaphysis is an incidental finding in a 25-year-old woman. The lesion has a thick sclerotic margin and there is a ground glass appearance to the matrix. There is a history of endocrine disturbance and several café-au-lait spots are evident on examination. Skeletal scintigraphy subsequently reveals multiple areas of increased activity within the skeleton. What is the most likely diagnosis?

A Gardner's syndrome
B Mazabraud's syndrome
C Maffucci's syndrome
D McCune-Albright
E Ollier's syndrome

Answer on page 126

QUESTION 35

A 19-year-old student returns to the UK following 4 months' travelling around the world. Radiographs reveal multiple oval areas of calcification, up to 1 cm in long axis, aligned in the direction of muscle fibres. What is the most likely diagnosis?

A Cysticercosis
B Dracunculus (guinea worm) infection
C Hydatid disease
D Loiasis
E Schistosomiasis

Answer on page 127

QUESTION 36

An 80-year-old man undergoes skeletal scintigraphy for multifocal skeletal pain, malaise and weight loss. The scintigram shows diffusely increased activity throughout the skeleton, with absent renal activity. What is the most likely diagnosis?

A Metastatic bladder cancer

B Metastatic colon cancer

C Metastatic gastric cancer

D Metastatic lung cancer

E Metastatic prostate cancer

Answer on page 127

QUESTION 37

A 20-year-old man is brought to the Emergency Department after diving into the shallow end of a swimming pool at a party. Witnesses describe a hyperflexion injury to the cervical spine. A fracture is identified on the lateral cervical radiograph. What is the most likely fracture configuration given the mechanism of injury?

A Anterior wedge fracture

B Burst fracture, with an anterior wedge fracture and a retropulsed fragment

C Fracture dislocation, with anterior dislocation of the more cranial vertebra and an avulsion fracture of the superoanterior margin of the more inferior vertebra

D Fracture of the pars interarticularis, in association with an avulsion fracture through the anteroinferior margin of the vertebra above

E Posterior elements fracture with anterior vertebral wedging

Answer on page 127

QUESTION 38

A young patient is newly diagnosed with diaphyseal aclasis. What would be the expected imaging findings?

A Multiple enchondromas
B Multiple enostoses
C Multiple osteochondromas
D Multiple osteomas
E Multiple osteoid osteomas

Answer on page 127

QUESTION 39

A 35-year-old woman injures her right foot during a fall whilst wearing high-heeled shoes. She is subsequently unable to weightbear, and the entire foot is bruised, swollen and tender. A radiograph of the foot initially appears normal, but the possibility of a Lisfranc fracture–dislocation prompts close attention to the tarsometatarsal alignment. What is the normal alignment in this area?

A Fifth metatarsal aligned with the lateral cuneiform
B First metatarsal aligned with the cuboid
C Fourth metatarsal aligned with the medial cuneiform
D Second metatarsal aligned with the middle cuneiform
E Third metatarsal aligned with the navicular

Answer on page 127

QUESTION 40

The unrestrained passenger of a vehicle involved in a high-energy road traffic accident is admitted with a 'hangman's fracture'. What is the most likely appearance on plain film?

A Fractures through the neural arch of C1
B Fractures through the neural arch of C2
C Fracture of the spinous process of C7
D Transverse fracture through the base of the dens
E Wedge compression fracture of an upper cervical vertebra

Answer on page 127

QUESTION 41

A 15-year-old boy is noted to have a solitary lytic lesion expanding the cortex of the proximal tibia. An MRI demonstrates multiple fluid levels. What is the most likely diagnosis?

A Aneurysmal bone cyst
B Enchondroma
C Giant cell tumour
D Ostcoblastoma
E Simple bone cyst

Answer on page 127

QUESTION 42

A 6-year-old boy is referred to the orthopaedic team with a limp. A pelvic radiograph reveals loss of height of the right femoral head, with fragmentation and sclerosis of the epiphysis. What is the most likely diagnosis?

A Developmental dysplasia of the hip
B Perthes' disease
C Septic arthritis
D Slipped upper femoral epiphysis
E Transient synovitis of the hip

Answer on page 128

QUESTION 43

A 65-year-old woman is referred for a pelvic radiograph to investigate intermittent right hip pain. The radiograph shows thin lucent lines within both inferior pubic rami. Which radiographic feature would support a diagnosis of osteoporotic fracture rather than osteomalacia?

A Callus formation
B Failure to extend across the entire width of the bone
C Sclerotic margin to lucencies
D Similar appearances within the proximal femora
E Symmetrical appearance

Answer on page 128

QUESTION 44

A young footballer has an MRI of the left knee following a recent injury. There is amorphous intermediate signal in the region of the anterior cruciate ligament and a bone contusion involving the articular surface of the lateral femoral condyle. In which other location is a bone contusion most likely?

A The anterolateral aspect of the tibia
B The anteromedial aspect of the tibia
C The central articular surface of the tibia
D The posterolateral aspect of the tibia
E The posteromedial aspect of the tibia

Answer on page 128

QUESTION 45

A radiograph of the thoracolumbar spine in a 75-year-old woman with a history of back pain shows an anterior wedge compression fracture of T11. What influence does this observation have on the likelihood of a subsequent fracture?

A Doubles the risk of another vertebral fracture
B Doubles the risk of a proximal femoral fracture
C Has little effect on the risk of a subsequent fragility fracture
D Triples the risk of another vertebral fracture
E Triples the risk of a proximal femoral fracture

Answer on page 128

QUESTION 46

A 50-year-old man has an MRI examination of his right shoulder. Which pattern of imaging features is compatible with a partial thickness supraspinatus tear?

A A gap between the distal and proximal portions of the tendon, with retraction of the proximal tendon

B Areas of increased signal on T1 and T2 images

C Areas of increased signal on T1 and T2 images, extending across the full thickness of the tendon

D Areas of intermediate signal on T1- and PD-weighted images, with low signal on T2w images

E Low signal on all sequences

Answer on page 128

QUESTION 47

A young man undergoes an MRI of the right knee due to clinical suspicion of an acute rupture of the ACL. The ACL is indistinct, and cannot be visualised in either the coronal or sagittal plane. Which additional features would be supportive of a diagnosis of ACL rupture?

A Bunching up of the PCL

B Oedema within the medial collateral ligament

C Posterior translation of the femur on the tibial condyles

D Straightening of the patellar ligament

E Tear of the medial meniscus

Answer on page 128

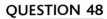

QUESTION 48

A 30-year-old man complains of intermittent painful swelling of his left knee over the past year. Radiographs show several small articular erosions, whilst subsequent MRI reveals foci of low T2/T2* signal intensity within the synovium. Which is the most likely diagnosis?

A Alkaptonuria

B Calcium pyrophosphate arthropathy

C Pigmented villonodular synovitis

D Psoriatic arthropathy

E Synovial chondromatosis

Answer on page 129

QUESTION 49

A 45-year-old man with hyperuricaemia is referred by the rheumatologists for an image-guided aspiration of a right ankle effusion. There is no previous history of note. A sample of the aspirate is sent for polarising light microscopy. What findings would confirm the clinical suspicion of gout?

A Rhomboid crystals

B Negatively birefringent needle shaped crystals

C Negatively birefringent rhomboid crystals

D Positively birefringent needle shaped crystals

E Positively birefringent rhomboid crystals

Answer on page 129

QUESTION 50

Which one of the following conditions is NOT a recognised component of the SAPHO spectrum?

A Arthritis
B Hyperostosis
C Osteomyelitis
D Pustulosis
E Synovitis

Answer on page 129

QUESTION 51

A 75-year-old diabetic man underwent a left below knee amputation 3 months ago for osteomyelitis of the distal tibia. Since then, he has experienced recurrent episodes of fever and malaise. MRI is contraindicated due to a metallic aortic valve. Which is the best investigation to exclude an occult focus of osteomyelitis?

A CT
B US
C Scintigraphy using gallium
D Scintigraphy using indium-labelled white cells
E Scintigraphy using technetium (Tc-99m) monodiphosphonate

Answer on page 129

QUESTION 52

A 30-year-old amateur footballer twists his right knee during a match, and is brought to the Emergency Medicine department with a painful swollen knee. Radiographs reveal an avulsion fracture closely related to the posterolateral tibial plateau, prompting an urgent MRI of the right knee. What are the most likely findings?

A Disruption of the extensor mechanism

B Rupture of the ACL

C Rupture of the PCL

D Tear of the medial meniscus

E Tear of the lateral collateral ligament

Answer on page 129

QUESTION 53

During an MRI examination of the shoulder, a 4-cm, well-defined structure is noted within the spinoglenoid notch, exhibiting high signal on T2w and low signal on T1w images. Which muscles should be carefully scrutinised for evidence of swelling or atrophy?

A Infraspinatus and supraspinatus

B Subscapularis and trapezius

C Supraspinatus and subscapularis

D Teres minor and infraspinatus

E Trapezius and teres minor

Answer on page 129

QUESTION 54

In relation to bone formation and turnover, defective osteoclastic function is a predominant feature of which disease?

A Osteomalacia
B Osteopetrosis
C Osteoporosis
D Paget's disease
E Rickets

Answer on page 130

QUESTION 55

An incidental finding on plain film is a 2-cm lucency within the diaphysis of the right humerus, which exhibits chondroid calcification. Which clinical or radiological feature would favour a diagnosis of chondrosarcoma rather than enchondroma?

A Age less than 20 years
B Circular, curvilinear or nodular calcific densities
C Periosteal reaction
D Slow growth
E Well-defined round or elliptical margin

Answer on page 130

QUESTION 56

A 40-year-old builder is admitted unconscious to the Emergency Department following an accident at work. Details of the accident are unclear, but one witness describes scaffolding collapsing. He undergoes an emergency CT head and cervical spine, which reveals lateral displacement of both the lateral masses of C1. How may such an injury be described?

A Atlanto-axial subluxation
B Clay shoveller's fracture
C Dens fracture
D Hangman's fracture
E Jefferson's fracture

Answer on page 130

QUESTION 57

A 20-year-old man complains of a 3-month history of pain from his left femur. The pain is of insidious onset and is worse at night. As part of his assessment, a bone scintigram is performed, which shows a corresponding area of abnormality in the left femoral shaft, characterised by a focus of very high activity surrounded by a diffuse area of modestly increased activity. What is the most likely diagnosis?

A Aneurysmal bone cyst
B Enostosis
C Enchondroma
D Osteoid osteoma
E Osteoma

Answer on page 130

QUESTION 58

An 18-year-old man experiences persistent symptoms following a fracture through the waist of the right scaphoid. Radiographs of the right scaphoid indicate non-union. An MRI is performed to assess the vascularity of the proximal pole. Which imaging features are consistent with a diagnosis of avascular necrosis?

A Bone marrow enhancement following administration of gadolinium

B High signal surrounding the fracture on T2w images

C High signal within the proximal pole on T1w images

D High signal within the proximal pole on STIR images

E Low signal within the proximal pole on T1w images

Answer on page 130

QUESTION 59

An 80-year-old diabetic man is admitted from the Emergency Department with clinical and radiographic features consistent with a septic arthritis of the right hip. There is no history of trauma or previous surgery. Initial blood cultures indicate a systemic bacteraemia. What is the most likely organism to be cultured?

A *Clostridium difficile*

B *Haemophilus influenzae*

C *Pseudomonas aeruginosa*

D *Staphylococcus aureus*

E *Streptococcus pneumoniae*

Answer on page 131

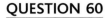

QUESTION 60

A 35-year-old man is brought to the Emergency Department following a fall from a motorcycle. The lateral cervical radiograph shows a well-marginated triangular area of bone at the anterosuperior margin of C5. The cortical margin of the adjacent vertebral body is smooth. The rest of the spine is normal. What is the most likely diagnosis?

A Avulsion of the anterior longitudinal ligament
B Limbus vertebra
C Schmorl's node
D Teardrop fracture of C5
E Unfused ring epiphysis

Answer on page 131

QUESTION 61

A 55-year-old lady, complaining of recent flattening of the longitudinal arch of the foot, is referred for an ultrasound examination of the left ankle. Which tendon should be the subject of particular scrutiny?

A Achilles tendon
B Flexor hallucis longus
C Peroneus longus
D Tibialis anterior
E Tibialis posterior

Answer on page 131

QUESTION 62

A 13-year-old boy is referred for radiographs of his hips following three weeks of right hip pain. What imaging features would support the diagnosis of slipped upper femoral epiphysis?

A Disruption of Klein's line

B Fragmentation of the femoral epiphysis

C Increased epiphyseal height

D Radiolucent subchondral fissure

E Sclerosis of the femoral head

Answer on page 131

QUESTION 63

A 55-year-old woman undergoes arthrography to investigate a 3-month history of pain and stiffness in her left shoulder, with particular limitation of external rotation. Only a few millilitres of contrast medium could be injected into the joint, before provoking discomfort. What other finding would be supportive of the diagnosis of adhesive capsulitis?

A Contrast medium opacifies the subacromial/subdeltoid bursa

B Decreased resistance to contrast injection

C Distended axillary recess

D Lymphatic filling

E Venous filling

Answer on page 131

QUESTION 64

The radiograph of a 40-year-old man with a painful knee shows multiple calcified loose bodies, each of similar size, within the joint. The joint space is preserved. What diagnosis is most likely?

A Calcium pyrophosphate arthropathy

B Gout

C Pigmented villonodular synovitis

D Rheumatoid arthritis

E Synovial osteochondromatosis

Answer on page 132

QUESTION 65

A 50-year-old man presents to the Emergency Department following an injury to his right hand. No fracture is detected on plain radiographs, but the second and third MCPJs appear abnormal, with joint space narrowing, subarticular cysts, hook-like osteophytes and flattening of the metacarpal heads. What is the most likely diagnosis?

A Alkaptonuria

B Gout

C Haemochromatosis

D Osteoarthritis

E Psoriatic arthritis

Answer on page 132

QUESTION 66

A 34-year-old man with chronic back pain is referred by his GP for thoracic and lumbar spine radiographs. The GP is concerned about the possibility of ankylosing spondylitis. Which radiological feature is atypical for ankylosing spondylitis, and might suggest an alternative diagnosis?

A Ankylosis of the apophyseal joints
B Anterior longitudinal ligament calcification
C Osteophyte formation
D Sclerosis of the anterior corners of the vertebrae
E Vertebral body squaring

Answer on page 132

QUESTION 67

A 70-year-old patient undergoes a staging CT for renal cell carcinoma, which shows ligamentous ossification extending from the fifth to ninth thoracic vertebrae. There is relative sparing of the left side of the vertebrae and disc space height is preserved. The apophyseal and sacroiliac joints appear normal. What is the most likely diagnosis?

A Ankylosing spondylitis
B Degenerative disc disease
C Diffuse idiopathic skeletal hyperostosis
D Metastatic disease
E Ossification of the posterior longitudinal ligament

Answer on page 132

QUESTION 68

A 50-year-old woman complains of painful swelling of the joints of
the hands and wrists. Radiographs show evidence of an erosive arthropathy.
Which radiological feature would favour a diagnosis of rheumatoid rather than
psoriatic arthritis?

A Early reduction in bone mineralisation
B Erosions of the terminal tufts of the distal phalanges
C Joint ankylosis
D Pencil-in-cup deformities of the middle phalanges
E Periosteal reaction

Answer on page 132

QUESTION 69

A 40-year-old tennis player undergoes an MRI following a 3-month history
of left ankle pain. The Achilles tendon has a convex anterior margin and
exhibits a small linear area of increased signal within the tendon on T2- and
T2*-weighted images. What is the most likely diagnosis?

A Achilles paratendonitis
B Achilles tendinosis
C Achilles tendinosis with complete tear
D Achilles tendinosis with cystic degeneration
E Achilles tendinosis with partial tear

Answer on page 133

QUESTION 70

A 30-year-old man undergoes an MRI examination of his left ankle, which shows a rounded mass within the pre-Achilles fat pad, with signal characteristics identical to adjacent muscle. Which anatomical variant could best account for these appearances?

A Accessory popliteus muscle

B Accessory soleus muscle

C Anomalous insertion of the gastrocnemius tendon

D Anomalous insertion of plantaris tendon

E Presence of peroneus quartus

Answer on page 133

QUESTION 71

A 9-year-old boy injures his right wrist playing football. The radiograph reveals a fracture extending through the epiphysis and into the metaphysis. How would this injury be classified in the Salter-Harris classification?

A Type I

B Type II

C Type III

D Type IV

E Type V

Answer on page 133

QUESTION 72

An 18-year-old man attends his general practitioner with a painful right knee. His radiograph shows a well-defined, lobular, lytic lesion within the proximal tibial epiphysis, extending into the metaphysis. There is a faintly sclerotic margin and no matrix calcification. What is the most likely diagnosis?

A Chondroblastoma

B Chondromyxoid fibroma

C Enchondroma

D Giant cell tumour

E Osteoid osteoma

Answer on page 133

QUESTION 73

A 50-year-old man has an MRI of his right shoulder for chronic shoulder pain The distal supraspinatus tendon displays intermediate signal intensity on T1w images and low signal intensity on T2w images. What is a possible explanation for these appearances?

A Chemical shift artefact

B Magic angle phenomenon

C Movement artefact in the frequency-encoding direction

D Movement artefact in the phase-encoding direction

E Susceptibility artefact from calcification

Answer on page 133

QUESTION 74

A series of neonatal radiographs reveal a narrow thorax with short ribs, square iliac wings with horizontal acetabular roofs, short sacrosciatic notches, progressive narrowing of the interpedicular distance and posterior scalloping of the vertebral bodies. What is the most likely diagnosis?

A Achondroplasia

B Campomelic dysplasia

C Cleidocranial dysplasia

D Ellis-van Creveld syndrome

E Morquio's syndrome

Answer on page 133

QUESTION 75

A 15-month-old boy is referred from his GP with a limp. Which radiological finding would be consistent with DDH?

A Accelerated epiphyseal ossification

B Decreased distance between the medial portion of the proximal femoral metaphysis and the pelvis

C Increased acetabular angle

D Inferolateral displacement of the femoral head in relation to Perkin's line

E Preservation of Shenton's line

Answer on page 134

QUESTION 76

A 35-year-old woman with back pain has radiographs taken of her lumbosacral spine. The frontal radiograph reveals narrowing of the right sacroiliac joint with significant periarticular sclerosis. The contralateral sacroiliac joint is normal. The lumbar spine is within normal limits for age. What is the most likely diagnosis?

A Ankylosing spondylitis

B Infection

C Osteitis condensans ilii

D Psoriatic arthropathy

E Reiter's syndrome

Answer on page 134

QUESTION 77

The skull radiograph of a 75-year-old man reveals a well-defined lytic area involving the frontal bone. A radiograph of the femur in the same patient shows a well-defined lucency extending from the articular surface to the diaphysis. The transition between lytic and normal bone is well defined and appears flame shaped. What is the most likely diagnosis?

A Acromegaly

B Fibrous dysplasia

C Myeloma

D Paget's disease

E Skeletal metastases

Answer on page 134

QUESTION 78

A 30-year-old man is admitted to hospital with chest pain. A chest radiograph demonstrates sclerosis of both humeral heads, pulmonary infiltrates and an elevated position of the splenic flexure immediately inferior to the left hemidiaphragm. What other associated imaging feature may be detected on the chest radiograph?

A A rib within a rib appearance

B Expansion of the head and neck of the ribs

C H-shaped vertebrae

D Paraspinal mass

E Posterior mediastinal mass

Answer on page 134

QUESTION 79

A young girl is brought to the Emergency Department with a painful right elbow following a fall. The radiograph reveals that the radial head is ossified. Which other structure should be visible?

A Capitellum

B Internal epicondyle

C Olecranon

D Lateral epicondyle

E Trochlea

Answer on page 135

QUESTION 80

A radiograph of the left knee of a 35-year-old man reveals a 3-cm lytic lesion sited eccentrically in the proximal tibia. It has a well-defined non-sclerotic margin, and extends to the tibial articular surface. What is the most likely diagnosis?

A Aneurysmal bone cyst
B Chondroblastoma
C Giant cell tumour
D Non-ossifying fibroma
E Osteoid osteoma

Answer on page 135

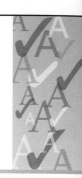

Musculoskeletal and Trauma

ANSWERS

QUESTION 1

ANSWER: E

Avulsion injuries occur at characteristic sites and are particularly common in children and adolescents.

Reference: *Grainger & Allison's* 5e, p 981.

QUESTION 2

ANSWER: B

Sclerosis of the margins of the epiphysis (Wimberger sign), metaphyseal (Pelcan) spurs, dense metaphyseal lines (white lines of Frankel) and exuberant periosteal reactions (secondary to recurrent subperiosteal bleeding) are features of scurvy. Expansion of the costochondral junctions results in the characteristic appearance of a rachitic rosary.

Reference: *Grainger & Allison's* 5e, pp 1104–1105; 1601.

QUESTION 3

ANSWER: E

Although eponymous classification of injuries is often criticised, many eponyms endure as succinct descriptions of fracture patterns, forcing the radiologist to remain aware of the more common eponymous injuries.
Reference: *Grainger & Allison's* 5e, pp 996–997.

QUESTION 4

ANSWER: B

Reference: *Grainger & Allison's* 5e, pp 1059–1060, Table 48.2 (p 1060) provides a useful summary of the likely sites of primary tumour.

QUESTION 5

ANSWER: E

Reference: *Grainger & Allison's* 5e, pp 980–981.

QUESTION 6

ANSWER: D

Reference: *Grainger & Allison's* 5e, pp 1063–1066.

QUESTION 7

ANSWER: A

Reference: *Grainger & Allison's* 5e, pp 1014–1023. Figure 46.104 (p 1016) gives a helpful summary of the pathomechanics of spinal injury.

QUESTION 8

ANSWER: C

Reference: *Grainger & Allison's* 5e, pp 974.

QUESTION 9

ANSWER: C

Skeletal metastases tend to involve the axial rather than appendicular skeleton, reflecting their predilection for bones containing red marrow. Metastases from bronchial carcinoma account for half of all peripheral metastases.

Reference: *Grainger & Allison's* 5e, pp 1060–1061.

QUESTION 10

ANSWER: D

Triplane fractures are injuries of adolescence, occurring around the time of epiphyseal fusion. Partial fusion of the growth plate results in complex fracture geometry following injury; typically, this includes a coronal metaphyseal fracture, a horizontal fracture through the physis and a sagittal epiphyseal fracture (eg Salter-Harris IV injury).

Tillaux fractures occur at a similar age, and are characterised by a horizontal fracture through the growth plate and a vertical epiphyseal fracture (Salter-Harris III injury).

Reference: *Grainger & Allison's* 5e, p 1618.

QUESTION 11

ANSWER: B

Reference: *Grainger & Allison's* 5e, p 1063 (Table 48.3 provides a concise summary).

QUESTION 12

ANSWER: C

Looser's zones represent areas of unmineralised osteoid and are pathognomonic of osteomalacia. The medial aspects of the proximal femora are typical sites for Looser's zones; other common sites include the pubic rami, ribs and the lateral border of the scapula.

Reference: *Grainger & Allison's* 5e, pp 1104–1105.

QUESTION 13

ANSWER: D

Reference: *Grainger & Allison's* 5e, pp 994–995.

QUESTION 14

ANSWER: A

Metaphyseal, rib, sternal and scapular fractures have a high specificity for non-accidental injury.

Reference: *Grainger & Allison's* 5e, p 1623.

QUESTION 15

ANSWER: B

Reference: *Grainger & Allison's* 5e, p 1141.

QUESTION 16

ANSWER: C

On a lateral radiograph, the length of the patellar tendon should equal the height of the patella, plus or minus 20%. Patella baja is associated with polio, juvenile chronic arthritis and achondroplasia.

Reference: *Grainger & Allison's* 5e, p 1140.

QUESTION 17

ANSWER: C

Reference: *Grainger & Allison's* 5e, p 1087.

QUESTION 18

ANSWER: E

The appearances are highly aggressive, and characteristic of osteosarcoma. The tumour matrix indicates a tumour of osseous rather than cartilaginous origin, making chondrosarcoma highly unlikely.

Reference: *Grainger & Allison's* 5e, pp 1066–1074, 1076.

QUESTION 19

ANSWER: C

The 'signet ring' appearance is due to rotatory subluxation of the scaphoid as a result of disruption of the scapholunate ligament.

Reference: *Grainger & Allison's* 5e, pp 998–999.

QUESTION 20

ANSWER: C

Reference: *Grainger & Allison's* 5e, pp 1148–1149.

QUESTION 21

ANSWER: B

Reference: *Grainger & Allison's* 5e, p 1100.

QUESTION 22

ANSWER: A

Reference: *Grainger & Allison's* 5e, p 1590 (Table 67.7 provides a concise summary).

QUESTION 23

ANSWER: E

An isolated lesser trochanter fracture is also highly suspicious for a pathological fracture.

Reference: *Grainger & Allison's* 5e, pp 1003–1004.

QUESTION 24

ANSWER: D

Reference: *Grainger & Allison's* 5e, p 1145.

QUESTION 25

ANSWER: E

Reference: *Grainger & Allison's* 5e, p 1147.

QUESTION 26

ANSWER: B

Kienboeck's disease describes lunate collapse as a result of vascular insufficiency and avascular necrosis. Avascular necrosis of the navicular is Köhler's disease whilst Freiberg's disease describes avascular necrosis of the second metatarsal head. Sever's disease relates to calcaneal apophysitis whilst Sinding-Larsen's disease is a cause of anterior knee pain in adolescents.

Reference: *Grainger & Allison's* 5e, p 1149.

QUESTION 27

ANSWER: E

Reference: *Grainger & Allison's* 5e, pp 1120–1130 (Table 50.7 on pp 1135–1136 provides a useful summary).

QUESTION 28

ANSWER: B

The detection, or exclusion, of osteomyelitis in the context of Charcot arthropathy is difficult. Bone marrow oedema is a feature of both infection and Charcot changes, but enhancement following gadolinium is suspicious for coexistent infection.

Reference: *Grainger & Allison's* 5e, p 1162.

QUESTION 29

ANSWER: D

Juxta-articular osteoporosis is a typical feature of haemophilic arthropathy, as a result of the periarticular hyperaemia associated with recurrent haemorrhage.

Reference: *Grainger & Allison's* 5e, pp 1118–1119.

QUESTION 30

ANSWER: B

Bone density can be measured in relation to an age and sex-matched population (Z score) or in relation to a population of young adults of the same sex (T score). The WHO defines osteoporosis as a T score less than −2.5, therefore relating bone mineral density to sex-matched peak bone mass.

Reference: *Grainger & Allison's* 5e, pp 1097–1099.

QUESTION 31

ANSWER: C

Reference: *Grainger & Allison's* 5e, p 1142.

QUESTION 32

ANSWER: D

Reference: *Grainger & Allison's* 5e, p 1134.

QUESTION 33

ANSWER: D

Infection and Langerhans cell histiocytosis (LCH) should be considered in the differential diagnosis of a permeative bone lesion in a child. Askin tumour is a rare primitive neuroectodermal tumour of the chest wall in children.

Reference: *Grainger & Allison's* 5e, pp 1074–1076.

QUESTION 34

ANSWER: D

McCune-Albright syndrome is characterised by polyostotic fibrous dysplasia, café-au-lait spots and endocrine disturbance (most commonly precocious puberty in girls). The rare association of polyostotic fibrous dysplasia and soft tissue mxyomas is Mazabraud's syndrome.

Reference: *Grainger & Allison's* 5e, pp 1037; 1041; 1054.

QUESTION 35

ANSWER: A

Reference: *Grainger & Allison's* 5e, pp 959–960.

QUESTION 36

ANSWER: E

Reference: *Grainger & Allison's* 5e, pp 1060–1061.

QUESTION 37

ANSWER: A

Reference: *Grainger & Allison's* 5e, p 1016 (Figure 46.104).

QUESTION 38

ANSWER: C

Reference: *Grainger & Allison's* 5e, pp 1035–1042.

QUESTION 39

ANSWER: D

Reference: *Grainger & Allison's* 5e, p 1012.

QUESTION 40

ANSWER: B

Reference: *Grainger & Allison's* 5e, pp 1015–1018.

QUESTION 41

ANSWER: A

Reference: *Grainger & Allison's* 5e, pp 1035–1055.

QUESTION 42

ANSWER: B

Reference: *Grainger & Allison's* 5e, p 1134.

QUESTION 43

ANSWER: A

Reference: *Grainger & Allison's* 5e, p 1105.

QUESTION 44

ANSWER: D

Reference: *Grainger & Allison's* 5e, p 1007.

QUESTION 45

ANSWER: B

Vertebral fractures are not only the most common fragility fracture, but also serve as powerful predictors of subsequent fracture. A vertebral fracture increases the likelihood of a further vertebral fracture fivefold, and doubles the risk of subsequent femoral neck fracture.

Reference: *Grainger & Allison's* 5e, pp 1088–1090 (Figure 49.4 (p 1089) provides a useful summary).

QUESTION 46

ANSWER: B

Reference: *Grainger & Allison's* 5e, pp 1145–1146.

QUESTION 47

ANSWER: A

Reference: *Grainger & Allison's* 5e, p 1139.

QUESTION 48

ANSWER: C

Reference: *Grainger & Allison's* 5e, pp 1132–1133.

QUESTION 49

ANSWER: B

Monosodium urate crystals are needle-shaped and strongly negatively birefringent under polarising light. Weakly positively birefringent rhomboid crystals are characteristic of calcium pyrophosphate dihydate deposition.

Reference: *Grainger & Allison's* 5e, p 1127.

QUESTION 50

ANSWER: A

Reference: *Grainger & Allison's* 5e, p 1164.

QUESTION 51

ANSWER: E

Although an indium-labelled white cell study is more specific, a bone scintigram using Tc-99m monodiphosphonate is a more sensitive test to exclude osteomyelitis.

Reference: *Grainger & Allison's* 5e, p 1159.

QUESTION 52

ANSWER: B

Reference: *Grainger & Allison's* 5e, pp 1005, 1139.

QUESTION 53

ANSWER: A

Reference: *Grainger & Allison's* 5e, pp 1147–1148.

QUESTION 54

ANSWER: B

Reference: *Grainger & Allison's* 5e, p 1084.

QUESTION 55

ANSWER: C

Outside the hands and feet, chondrosarcoma is five times more common than enchondroma.

Reference: *Grainger & Allison's* 5e, pp 1035–1040.

QUESTION 56

ANSWER: E

Reference: *Grainger & Allison's* 5e, pp 1016–1017.

QUESTION 57

ANSWER: D

Reference: *Grainger & Allison's* 5e, pp 1035–1055, particularly pp 1041–1042.

QUESTION 58

ANSWER: E

Low signal on T1 reflects death of the adipocytes. The combination of low signal on T1w images and low or intermediate signal on T2w images accurately predicts avascular necrosis.

Reference: *Grainger & Allison's* 5e, p 1150.

QUESTION 59

ANSWER: D

Streptococcus pneumoniae and *Haemophilus influenzae* are potential causes of primary bacteraemia and haematogenous infection of joints, but substantially less common than *Staphylococcus aureus*.

Reference: *Grainger & Allison's* 5e, p 1153.

QUESTION 60

ANSWER: B

Reference: *Grainger & Allison's* 5e, p 1024.

QUESTION 61

ANSWER: E

Reference: *Grainger & Allison's* 5e, p 1144.

QUESTION 62

ANSWER: A

Klein's line is drawn along the lateral border of the femoral neck and normally intersects roughly a sixth of the femoral epiphysis. Subchondral fissuring (crescent sign), epiphyseal collapse, fragmentation and sclerosis are all features of Perthes' disease.

Reference: *Grainger & Allison's* 5e, pp 1592–1593.

QUESTION 63

ANSWER: D

Reference: *Grainger & Allison's* 5e, pp 1133–1134.

QUESTION 64

ANSWER: E

Reference: *Grainger & Allison's* 5e, p 1133.

QUESTION 65

ANSWER: C

Reference: *Grainger & Allison's* 5e, p 1130.

QUESTION 66

ANSWER: C

Syndesmophytes, rather than osteophytes, are characteristic features of ankylosing spondylitis. They are differentiated from osteophytes by their vertical orientation, as they represent ossification of the outer border of the annulus fibrosus. Progression and maturation of the syndesmophytes result in a 'bamboo spine'.

Reference: *Grainger & Allison's* 5e, pp 1125–1126.

QUESTION 67

ANSWER: C

Reference: *Grainger & Allison's* 5e, p 1118.

QUESTION 68

ANSWER: A

Juxta-articular osteopenia is one of the earliest radiographic abnormalities in rheumatoid arthritis, distinguishing it from psoriatic arthropathy, in which bone mineral density is preserved until late in the disease process.

Reference: *Grainger & Allison's* 5e, pp 1120–1123 (Table 50.7 (pp 1135–1136) provides a useful summary).

QUESTION 69

ANSWER: E

Reference: *Grainger & Allison's* 5e, pp 1142–1143.

QUESTION 70

ANSWER: B

Reference: *Grainger & Allison's* 5e, p 1144.

QUESTION 71

ANSWER: D

Reference: *Grainger & Allison's* 5e, p 1613 (Figure 68.5 provides a concise summary).

QUESTION 72

ANSWER: A

Reference: *Grainger & Allison's* 5e, pp 1035–1055.

QUESTION 73

ANSWER: B

The magic angle phenomenon refers to the increased signal observed on sequences with a short echo time (eg T1w, proton density (PD)) within tissues containing parallel unidirectional collagen fibres, when such fibres are at an angle of 55° to the main magnetic field. It is of particular relevance in shoulder MR, where it may mimic supraspinatus tendinosis.

Reference: *Grainger & Allison's* 5e, p 1145.

QUESTION 74

ANSWER: A

The iliac wings in Morquio's syndrome are characteristically flared rather than square.

Reference: *Grainger & Allison's* 5e, pp 1567–1588 (Table 67.4 provides a useful summary).

QUESTION 75

ANSWER: C

Reference: *Grainger & Allison's* 5e, pp 1588–1592 (Figure 67.29 illustrates the imaging features of DDH).

QUESTION 76

ANSWER: B

Infection is the commonest cause of unilateral sacroiliitis, and TB should be considered as a possible organism. Ankylosing spondylitis and osteitis condensans ilii have symmetrical appearances, whilst Reiter's syndrome is bilateral (but asymmetric). Psoriatic arthropathy produces bilateral disease, which is symmetrical in most cases.

References: *Grainger & Allison's* 5e, pp 1122–1128, 1161.
Chapman S, Nakielny R. *Aids to Radiological Differential Diagnosis*, 5th edition (Edinburgh: Saunders, 2003), p 58.

QUESTION 77

ANSWER: D

Paget's disease is a condition of uncertain aetiology characterised by increased turnover and excessive remodelling of bone. Osteoporosis circumscripta and advancing flame-shaped lucencies within long bones are features characteristic of active osteolytic disease. Inactive disease is characterised by widespread sclerosis: cotton wool sclerosis in the skull, enlarged ivory vertebrae with cortical thickening and coarsened thick trabeculae within the long bones. Paget's disease may be complicated by fractures, accelerated osteoarthritis and sarcomatous change.

Reference: Chapman & Nakielny R, *Aids to Radiological Differential Diagnosis*, pp 459–460.

QUESTION 78

ANSWER C

In sickle cell disease, infarction of the central endplates of the vertebrae results in H-shaped or codfish vertebrae. Rib changes, paraspinal and posterior mediastinal masses are manifestations of extramedullary haematopoiesis in thalassaemia.

Reference: *Grainger & Allison's* 5e, pp 1603–1604.

QUESTION 79

ANSWER: A

Reference: *Grainger & Allison's* 5e, pp 1613–1614.

QUESTION 80

ANSWER: C

Reference: *Grainger & Allison's* 5e, pp 1046–1047.

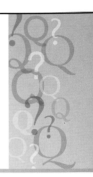

MODULE 3

Gastrointestinal

QUESTIONS

QUESTION 1

A 53-year-old woman is seen in the general surgical outpatient clinic. She attended her GP with a 1-month history of upper abdominal pain and was found to have a palpable, firm mass in the epigastrium. An upper gastrointestinal (GI) endoscopy is normal and the surgical team request a contrast-enhanced CT of the abdomen. This demonstrates a multicystic mass in the pancreas. Which findings would make a mucinous cystic tumour more likely than a serous cystadenoma?

A Central stellate calcification is present within the lesion.
B The mass contains 12 separate cysts.
C The smallest cystic component measures 28 mm in diameter.
D The patient has a known diagnosis of von Hippel-Lindau disease.
E The tumour is located in the head of the pancreas.

Answer on page 189

QUESTION 2

A 54-year-old man with hepatitis B cirrhosis attends the hepatology outpatient clinic. The patient's serum alpha fetoprotein level is found to be significantly elevated, having been normal 6 months ago. An abdominal ultrasound demonstrates a new 3-cm lesion in the right lobe of liver and a diagnosis of hepatocellular carcinoma (HCC) is suspected. Which one of the following statements is correct regarding HCC?

A Brain metastases are hypovascular and calcified.

B HCC derives its blood supply primarily from the hepatic artery.

C Portal vein invasion is more suggestive of a liver metastasis than HCC.

D Small HCC (< 1 cm) are typically heterogeneous and hyperechoic on US.

E The bony skeleton is the most common site for distant metastases.

Answer on page 189

QUESTION 3

A 22-year-old man is brought to the Emergency Department with a 2-day history of increasingly severe upper abdominal pain and vomiting. He has not opened his bowels for 24 hours but has passed flatus. The patient is usually fit and well but admits to consuming 100 units of alcohol per week. Initial laboratory investigations show an elevated white cell count and a significantly raised serum amylase. An abdominal radiograph is performed and demonstrates a single segment of dilated small bowel in the central abdomen. What name is given to this radiographic finding?

A Arrowhead sign

B Bird of prey sign

C Football sign

D Ranson's sign

E Sentinel loop sign

Answer on page 190

QUESTION 4

A 72-year-old man presents to his GP with increasing dyspepsia and weight loss. He has not experienced any other GI symptoms and physical examination is unremarkable. A barium meal is performed with the administration of intravenous Buscopan. The oesophagus is normal in appearance but a 'bull's eye' lesion is noted in the gastric mucosa. Which one of the following is not a recognised cause of this appearance?

A Gastric carcinoma

B Gastrointestinal stromal tumour (GIST)

C Magenstrasse

D Melanoma metastases

E Neurofibromatosis

Answer on page 190

QUESTION 5

A 19-year-old female student presents with acute abdominal pain, elevated CRP and a low-grade temperature. On clinical examination, there is tenderness to light palpation in the right iliac fossa and the patient is febrile. A graded compression ultrasound examination is performed. Which one of the following statements is true?

A A transverse appendiceal diameter of 5 mm is diagnostic of acute appendicitis.

B The finding of a pelvic fluid collection makes a diagnosis of acute appendicitis unlikely.

C The presence of hyperechoic fat in the right iliac fossa makes a diagnosis of acute appendicitis unlikely.

D The sensitivity of graded compression ultrasound in suspected acute appendicitis is 75–90%.

E The specificity of graded compression ultrasound in suspected acute appendicitis is 35–50%.

Answer on page 190

QUESTION 6

A 42-year-old man presents to the Emergency Department with a 7-day history of severe bloody diarrhoea and abdominal pain. He has previously been fit and well with no significant medical history. On examination, the patient is dehydrated with generalized abdominal tenderness but no clinical evidence of peritonism. An abdominal radiograph is performed. Which radiographic finding would be most suggestive of a toxic megacolon?

A Caecum measuring 4.5 cm in diameter

B Multiple mucosal islands in a dilated transverse colon

C Pseudodiverticulae in the descending colon

D Thickened haustrae throughout the entire colon

E 'Thumbprinting' of the transverse and descending colon

Answer on page 191

QUESTION 7

A 54-year-old woman attends a well woman clinic and is found to have abnormal liver function tests. She is referred to the hepatology outpatient clinic and an abdominal ultrasound is performed. This demonstrates diffuse increased reflectivity of the liver parenchyma but no focal parenchymal abnormality. The hepatology team request an ultrasound-guided percutaneous liver biopsy. Which statement is true regarding this procedure?

A Ten to 20% of complications occur in the first 2 hours post procedure.

B Ascites is an absolute contraindication to percutaneous liver biopsy.

C Mortality rate is 1 in 500.

D Over 90% of complications occur in the first 24 hours post procedure.

E There is no increased risk of complications with malignant liver lesions.

Answer on page 191

QUESTION 8

A 26-year-old man presents to the Emergency Department with acute epigastric pain and vomiting. The serum amylase is found to be markedly elevated and the patient is treated for acute pancreatitis. A contrast-enhanced CT of the abdomen is subsequently performed and demonstrates calcification throughout the pancreas. Bilateral renal calculi are also noted. What is the most likely underlying diagnosis?

A Hereditary pancreatitis

B Hyperparathyroidism

C Hypoparathyroidism

D Mucinous cystadenocarcinoma

E Multiple pancreatic pseudocysts

Answer on page 191

QUESTION 9

A 53-year-old man has a history of type 2 diabetes mellitus and nonalcoholic steatohepatitis. He complains of weight loss and malaise; therefore an abdominal ultrasound is performed. This demonstrates a 2-cm focal lesion in the liver parenchyma. Which additional findings would be most consistent with an area of focal fatty sparing in hepatic steatosis?

A There is avid enhancement of the lesion on contrast-enhanced ultrasound.

B The focal area is of increased echogenicity, compared to that of the surrounding liver.

C The lesion has a geographic margin and is of reduced echogenicity compared to that of the surrounding liver.

D The lesion is hypoechoic with vessels displaced around its margins.

E The lesion is in the gallbladder fossa and is associated with segmental intrahepatic biliary dilatation.

Answer on page 191

QUESTION 10

A 29-year-old man presents with a 6-month history of dysphagia, associated with retrosternal pain. A barium swallow demonstrates a markedly dilated oesophagus containing food debris. There is a smooth narrowing of the distal oesophagus with barium intermittently spurting into the stomach. What is the most likely diagnosis?

A Oesophageal achalasia
B Oesophageal leiomyoma
C Paraoesophageal hiatus hernia.
D Peptic oesophageal stricture
E Squamous cell carcinoma of the oesophagus

Answer on page 192

QUESTION 11

A 68-year-old woman presents with malaise and abdominal pain and is found to have abnormal liver function tests. An abdominal ultrasound identifies multiple hyperechoic lesions in the liver and contrast-enhanced CT of the abdomen demonstrates that these are hypervascular liver metastases. Given the CT findings, what is the most likely underlying diagnosis?

A Carcinoid
B Lymphoma
C Non-small-cell lung cancer
D Ovarian epithelial carcinoma
E Transitional cell carcinoma (TCC) of bladder

Answer on page 192

QUESTION 12

A 35-year-old pregnant woman (28 weeks gestation) presents to her GP with right upper quadrant abdominal pain and is found to have abnormal liver function tests. An abdominal ultrasound is performed and demonstrates a diffusely hyperechoic liver with a discrete 4-cm hypoechoic lesion in the right lobe. An MRI is performed 3 weeks later, showing that the liver lesion has increased in size, now measuring 7 cm diameter. The lesion is isointense on in-phase T1w images, losing signal on out-of-phase images. Following intravenous gadolinium there is immediate and intense enhancement with early washout. What is the most likely diagnosis?

A Choriocarcinoma
B Focal nodular hyperplasia
C Hepatic adenoma
D Liver haemangioma
E Metastatic breast cancer

Answer on page 192

QUESTION 13

A 59-year-old man undergoes surgical resection of a rectal tumour. A contrast-enhanced CT of the abdomen is performed 3 months later and demonstrates a new, solitary 3-cm liver metastasis. The lesion lies inferior to the level of the left and right portal veins and posterior to the right hepatic vein. The remainder of the CT examination is unremarkable and the patient is assessed for surgical resection of the liver lesion. Which segment of the liver does the liver metastasis lie in?

A Segment 4b
B Segment 5
C Segment 6
D Segment 7
E Segment 8

Answer on page 192

QUESTION 14

A 74-year-old man presents with an 8-week history of altered bowel habit and rectal bleeding. A flexible sigmoidoscopy demonstrates a malignant stricture in the rectum and biopsies confirm rectal adenocarcinoma. An MRI is performed and shows an annular neoplasm at 12 cm. The mass invades 4 mm beyond the rectal wall into the perirectal fat and infiltrates the peritoneal reflection anteriorly. There is a small volume of free peritoneal fluid. What is the radiological T stage?

A TX

B T1

C T2

D T3

E T4

Answer on page 193

QUESTION 15

A 38-year-old woman receives an orthotopic liver transplant for chronic liver failure due to primary biliary cirrhosis. The patient's liver enzyme levels become markedly elevated after 24 hours and her clinical condition deteriorates. An abdominal ultrasound is performed with Doppler evaluation of the hepatic vessels. Given the clinical history, which vascular complication is most likely to have occurred?

A Arterioportal fistula

B IVC thrombosis

C Hepatic artery stenosis

D Hepatic artery thrombosis

E Portal vein thrombosis

Answer on page 193

QUESTION 16

A 37-year-old man presents to his GP with increasing right upper quadrant pain. On examination, he is afebrile with right upper quadrant tenderness and fullness. An abdominal ultrasound is performed and demonstrates a 5-cm diameter cystic lesion in the right lobe of liver. The mass contains multiple septations with a large cyst centrally and multiple small cystic spaces peripherally. Echogenic debris is seen within the cystic lesion and alters in position when the patient lies on his side. From the clinical and sonographic details, what is the most likely diagnosis?

A Amoebic abscess
B Hydatid cyst
C Pyogenic liver abscess
D Simple liver cyst
E Solitary metastasis

Answer on page 193

QUESTION 17

A 48-year-old woman is noted to have elevated liver enzymes on blood tests performed by her GP. She attends the radiology department and an abdominal ultrasound is performed. This demonstrates moderate diffuse fatty infiltration of the liver and thickening of the wall of the gallbladder fundus. Hyperechoic foci are seen in the gallbladder wall with 'ring-down' reverberation artefacts. There is no acoustic shadowing. What is the most likely diagnosis?

A Adenomyomatosis
B Chronic cholecystitis
C Multiple gallstones with acute cholecystitis
D Porcelain gallbladder
E Xanthogranulomatous cholecystitis

Answer on page 194

QUESTION 18

A 68-year-old man presents to his GP with a 1-month history of epigastric pain, vomiting and mild weight loss. Examination is unremarkable and the patient is referred for an upper gastrointestinal endoscopy. This demonstrates mild gastritis with biopsies positive for *Helicobacter pylori* and he is commenced on eradication therapy. Three months later, the symptoms have persisted and the patient has lost 5 kg in weight. A double contrast barium meal is performed and reveals a shallow ulcer on the lesser curve of the stomach. Which additional finding would make the ulcer more likely to be benign than malignant?

A Hampton's line is present.

B Nodular mucosal folds stop at the edge of the lesion.

C The ulcer does not extend beyond the gastric wall.

D The ulcer has an irregular margin.

E The ulcer measures 40 mm in size.

Answer on page 194

QUESTION 19

A 42-year-old man has type 1 diabetes mellitus. Despite intensive medical management, the patient's glycaemic control remains problematic and he receives a cadaveric pancreatic transplant with the pancreatic graft anastomosed to the right common iliac artery. Four days following surgery, the clinical team are concerned about the pancreatic graft function and request radiological assessment for post-transplant complications. Which one of the following statements is true regarding pancreatic transplant imaging?

A In acute rejection, the pancreatic graft is small and hyperechoic on ultrasound.

B Pancreatic exocrine secretions often drain into the urinary bladder.

C Radionuclide imaging with Tc-99m-pertechnetate is the most sensitive way of detecting acute pancreatic rejection.

D Surgical complications are more common following renal transplantation than pancreatic transplantation.

E Transplant pancreatitis is very rare in the first 48 hours post surgery.

Answer on page 194

QUESTION 20

A 49-year-old man presents to his GP with increasing dysphagia and weight loss. Upper gastrointestinal endoscopy reveals a tumour in the distal oesophagus and biopsies confirm oesophageal adenocarcinoma. The patient undergoes a contrast-enhanced CT of the chest and abdomen which shows mucosal thickening in the distal oesophagus but no other abnormality.
An endoscopic ultrasound is performed and shows that the tumour infiltrates through the muscularis propria and adventitia but does not extend beyond the serosa. A round 13-mm peritumoral node is noted. From this information, what is the TNM staging of this tumour?

A T2 N0 M0
B T2 N1 M0
C T3 N0 M0
D T3 N1 M0
E T4 N1 M0

Answer on page 194

QUESTION 21

A male patient is referred to the on-call surgical team with a 3-day history of generalised abdominal pain and vomiting. The patient has not opened his bowels for 2 days. Examination reveals a distended abdomen with increased bowel sounds. An abdominal radiograph is performed and demonstrates a large dilated loop of large bowel with several loops of dilated small bowel centrally. Which other feature would make a diagnosis of caecal volvulus more likely than that of sigmoid volvulus?

A Haustrae are visible in the gas-filled viscus.
B The apex of the viscus lies in the left upper quadrant.
C The patient is 75 years old.
D The patient is in long-term institutional care.
E The viscus rises above the level of the T10 vertebral body.

Answer on page 195

QUESTION 22

A 59-year-old man is diagnosed with squamous cell carcinoma of the lower oesophagus. A contrast-enhanced CT of the chest and abdomen demonstrates a right paratracheal lymph node that measures 9 mm in the short axis, with no evidence of distant metastases. The patient is considered for surgery and a PET-CT examination is performed. The PET-CT demonstrates no uptake in the right paratracheal lymph node, but there is symmetrical uptake of 18-FDG in both supraclavicular areas. What is the most likely explanation for this finding?

A Brown adipose tissue

B Paraneoplastic polymyositis

C Recent trauma

D Recent viral upper respiratory tract infection

E Uncontrolled diabetes mellitus

Answer on page 195

QUESTION 23

A 52-year-old female patient is under the care of a rheumatologist with a diagnosis of diffuse scleroderma. She presents to her GP with vomiting, intermittent abdominal pain and reduced bowel habit. An abdominal radiograph demonstrates several loops of gas-filled bowel but there is no evidence of mechanical obstruction. A barium follow-through examination is performed. In view of the clinical history, what are the most likely findings?

A Dilated small bowel with increased number of valvulae conniventes

B Extraluminal mass in the ileum, causing ulceration and a shouldered stricture

C Long irregular ileal stricture with antimesenteric mucosal thickening

D Nodular thickening of the valvulae conniventes of the duodenum only

E Short stricture in the terminal ileum with 'cobblestoning' of the mucosa

Answer on page 195

QUESTION 24

A 23-year-old woman complains of episodes of diarrhoea and rectal bleeding. Her father died of colorectal cancer aged 39. A double contrast barium enema is performed and demonstrates more than one hundred small polyps, measuring up to 5 mm in size, throughout the colon. An upper GI endoscopy demonstrates multiple polypoid lesions in the stomach and duodenum. What is the most likely diagnosis?

A Carcinoid syndrome

B Familial adenomatous polyposis

C Hereditary non-polyposis colorectal cancer

D Juvenile polyposis

E Peutz-Jeghers syndrome

Answer on page 195

QUESTION 25

A 78-year-old man has myelodysplastic syndrome and requires frequent blood transfusions. He develops progressively abnormal liver function tests and a grossly elevated ferritin level. An MRI of the liver is performed using breath hold half Fourier single shot spin echo T2w images. Which finding would make a diagnosis of haemosiderosis (iron overload from recurrent blood transfusion) more likely than haemochromatosis?

A Increased T2 signal in the liver only

B Increased T2 signal in the liver and spleen

C Reduced T2 signal in the liver only

D Reduced T2 signal in the liver and spleen

E Reduced T2 signal in the spleen only

Answer on page 196

QUESTION 26

A 31-year-old woman develops mild acute pancreatitis and is managed conservatively. It is her third episode of pancreatitis but there is no history of excess alcohol consumption and an abdominal ultrasound is normal. Magnetic resonance cholangiopancreatography (MRCP) is performed and is reported as showing evidence of pancreas divisum. Which one of the following findings is likely to have been present on MRCP?

A A 3-cm cystic structure in the head of the pancreas

B An accessory pancreatic duct passing around the duodenum

C The common bile duct draining into the minor papilla

D The dorsal pancreatic duct (duct of Santorini) draining into the minor papilla

E The ventral pancreatic duct draining into the minor papilla

Answer on page 196

QUESTION 27

A 47-year-old woman presents with a 2-day history of lower abdominal pain and reduced bowel habit. Dilated loops of small bowel are evident on an abdominal radiograph and a barium small bowel follow-through examination is performed. This demonstrates a stricture in a pelvic loop of small bowel. The patient's symptoms improve on conservative management and further history reveals pelvic radiotherapy for cervical cancer 21 years ago. Which one of the following statements is true regarding radiation enteritis?

A Acute symptoms following radiotherapy are a poor predictor of chronic enteritis.

B The proximal jejunum is the most common site of small bowel involvement.

C There is characteristic dilatation of affected small bowel in chronic radiation enteritis.

D There is flattening of the valvulae conniventes in the acute stage.

E There is typically 'cobblestoning' of the small bowel mucosa.

Answer on page 196

QUESTION 28

A 22-year-old woman presents to her GP with a 4-month history of increasing right upper quadrant pain. An abdominal ultrasound is performed and demonstrates a 6-cm solid lesion of increased reflectivity in segment 6 of the liver. A contrast-enhanced CT of the liver is performed and demonstrates that the lesion enhances moderately and has a lobulated margin. Which additional finding would make a diagnosis of fibrolamellar carcinoma more likely than that of focal nodular hyperplasia (FNH)?

A A hyperechoic central scar

B A preexisting history of chronic liver disease

C Delayed enhancement of a central scar

D Punctuate calcification in the lesion

E The patient is taking the combined oral contraceptive pill

Answer on page 197

QUESTION 29

A 35-year-old woman is referred to the Radiology Department following the birth of her first child. The baby was delivered 8 days post-term and was a vaginal delivery following a prolonged labour and episiotomy. Two months later, the patient continues to experience faecal incontinence and an anal sphincter tear is suspected. Which investigation would be most useful to demonstrate anal sphincter damage?

A Barium evacuation proctogram

B CT colonography

C CT with rectal contrast media

D Endoanal ultrasound

E MRI of the pelvis with a body coil

Answer on page 197

QUESTION 30

A 33-year-old woman presents to her GP with a one year history of intermittent rectal bleeding. She experiences regular episodes of fresh blood per rectum with associated lower abdominal pain, lasting several days at a time. A flexible sigmoidoscopy is normal. A double contrast barium enema is performed and demonstrates an irregular appearance of the anterior wall of the sigmoid colon with mild extrinsic mass effect. What is the most likely diagnosis?

A Carcinoma of the sigmoid colon

B Endometriosis

C Pelvic lipomatosis

D Radiation enteritis

E Solitary rectal ulcer syndrome

Answer on page 197

QUESTION 31

A 52-year-old man undergoes a thoracoabdominal oesophagectomy for squamous cell carcinoma of the mid oesophagus. The patient has an uncomplicated postoperative recovery and is discharged home. Four weeks later, a chest radiograph is performed. Which one finding would be unexpected on this chest radiograph?

A Absence of right 5th rib posteriorly

B Retrocardiac air:fluid level

C Right paramediastinal soft tissue density mass

D Moderate left hydropneumothorax

E Vertical staple line in the mediastinum

Answer on page 197

QUESTION 32

A 59-year-old man presents to his GP with a 3-day history of right upper quadrant pain and vomiting. There is a past medical history of ischaemic heart disease and type 2 diabetes mellitus. An abdominal ultrasound demonstrates thickening of the gallbladder wall and pericholecystic fluid, but no gallstones. The patient deteriorates clinically with elevation of white cell count and CRP levels. A repeat ultrasound 3 days later demonstrates a bright echogenic area in the gallbladder fundus with acoustic shadowing. What is the most likely diagnosis?

A Adenomyomatosis

B Emphysematous cholecystitis

C Gallbladder carcinoma

D Mirizzi syndrome

E Porcelain gallbladder

Answer on page 198

QUESTION 33

A 48-year-old man presents to his GP with epigastric pain, diarrhoea and weight loss over a period of 6 months. Laboratory investigations reveal a reduced serum albumin, and a contrast-enhanced CT of the abdomen demonstrates diffuse thickening of the gastric mucosa. A double contrast barium meal examination is performed and shows markedly thickened mucosal folds in the gastric body with sparing of the gastric antrum. The mucosal folds alter in size and position during the examination. What is the most likely diagnosis?

A Eosinophilic gastritis

B Gastric lymphoma

C Infiltrative gastric adenocarcinoma (linitis plastica)

D Ménétrier's disease

E Organoaxial gastric volvulus

Answer on page 198

QUESTION 34

A 46-year-old woman from Bangladesh is being treated for pulmonary tuberculosis. Despite anti-tuberculosis chemotherapy, she develops increasing fevers with abdominal discomfort and distension. An abdominal and pelvic ultrasound demonstrates a moderate volume of peritoneal free fluid, and a contrast-enhanced CT of the abdomen and pelvis is performed. What are the likely findings on CT?

A A mixed solid:cystic ovarian mass with serosal deposits on the liver and spleen

B Ascites with enlarged mesenteric lymph nodes containing high attenuation centres

C Gastric wall thickening extending into the spleen with enlarged coeliac axis lymph nodes and ascites

D Peritoneal nodularity with high density ascites

E Portal vein thrombosis with ascites

Answer on page 198

QUESTION 35

A 56-year-old woman presents to her GP with a 4-week history of lethargy and increasing jaundice. She is previously fit and well with no history of biliary or liver disease. An abdominal ultrasound is performed and demonstrates moderate intrahepatic biliary dilatation. Which feature in the patient's medical history would significantly increase the risk of cholangiocarcinoma?

A Drug history of regular nonsteroidal anti-inflammatory drug (NSAID) usage

B Past medical history of giardiasis 2 years ago

C Past medical history of ulcerative colitis

D Jaundice associated with right upper quadrant pain

E Patient allergic to iodinated contrast media

Answer on page 198

QUESTION 36

A 49-year-old man develops weight loss, upper abdominal pain and three episodes of vomiting fresh red blood. Subsequent upper gastrointestinal endoscopy reveals a distal gastric adenocarcinoma. The patient undergoes a surgical procedure to resect the tumour, but develops increasing epigastric pain and fever 4 days later. An upper GI contrast study is performed. Which one of the following statements is true regarding this examination?

A A partial distal gastrectomy with gastrojejunostomy (Billroth II procedure) involves an end-to-end anastomosis.

B Control images prior to contrast administration are not indicated in this setting.

C If a water-soluble contrast examination appears normal, barium can be used as it has a higher sensitivity in identifying anastomotic leaks.

D The oesophago-gastric junction is the most common site for perforation and contrast leaks.

E Thickening of the mucosa at the surgical anastomosis with delayed gastric emptying is most likely due to residual gastric tumour.

Answer on page 199

QUESTION 37

A 47-year-old woman with obstructive jaundice undergoes an MRCP examination. This demonstrates a smooth stricture in the mid-common duct with associated moderate intrahepatic biliary dilatation. The stricture is caused by extrinsic compression from a round filling defect within the cystic duct. What is the diagnosis?

A Acute bacterial cholangitis

B Gallbladder carcinoma

C Mirizzi syndrome

D Postinflammatory biliary stricture

E Primary sclerosing cholangitis (PSC)

Answer on page 199

QUESTION 38

A 56-year-old woman presents with a 4-day history of right upper quadrant pain and vomiting. She describes a previous episode one year ago that resolved after a few days. On examination, she is very tender in the right upper quadrant with guarding on deep palpation during inspiration. Laboratory investigations reveal elevated white cell count and CRP but normal liver function tests and an abdominal ultrasound is performed. What are the most likely ultrasound findings?

A Hypoechoic mass in the pancreatic head with common bile duct measuring 14 mm and pancreatic duct measuring 6 mm in diameter

B Nodular liver surface, mixed reflectivity liver texture and ascites

C Severe intrahepatic duct dilatation with no cause identified

D Several large gallstones with gallbladder wall measuring 5 mm and a rim of pericholecystic fluid

E Several small gallstones with gallbladder wall thickness of 2 mm

Answer on page 199

QUESTION 39

A 42-year-old man is admitted to hospital with acute abdominal pain. There is a significant medical history of polycythaemia rubra vera, for which the patient undergoes regular venesection. On examination, there is right upper quadrant tenderness and hepatomegaly. Liver function tests are acutely elevated and the patient's condition deteriorates. A catheter angiogram is performed to assess the major hepatic vessels and shows a 'spider's web' appearance within the liver. What is the diagnosis?

A Budd Chiari syndrome

B Capillary haemangioma

C Hereditary haemorrhagic telangiectasia (HHT)

D Portal vein thrombosis

E Spontaneous hepatic haematoma

Answer on page 199

QUESTION 40

A 74-year-old woman is referred to the hepatology outpatient clinic with persistently abnormal liver function tests. There is a past medical history of myocardial infarction, atrial fibrillation and hypertension, but no previous history of liver disease. On abdominal ultrasound, the liver appears normal with antegrade portal venous flow demonstrated. A CT of the abdomen is performed and the mean density of the liver is 86 Hounsfield Units (HU) precontrast. What is the most likely diagnosis?

A Amiodarone therapy

B Chronic Budd Chiari syndrome

C Chronic hepatitis B

D Diffuse fatty infiltration

E Wilson's disease

Answer on page 200

QUESTION 41

A 68-year-old man presents to his GP with weight loss and jaundice. Liver function tests demonstrate obstructive jaundice and an abdominal ultrasound shows mild intrahepatic biliary dilatation with a common bile duct measuring 12 mm in diameter. In the pancreatic head, a 3-cm hypoechoic mass is present. An ERCP is performed with insertion of a plastic stent and brushings confirm a pancreatic ductal adenocarcinoma. A triple-phase (precontrast, arterial and portal venous) multidetector CT of the pancreas is performed. Which finding would indicate a nonresectable pancreatic tumour?

A Enhancing pancreatic parenchyma between the tumour and superior mesenteric vein

B The pancreatic duct dilated to 6 mm

C The presence of a 5-mm coeliac axis lymph node

D The tumour has invaded the duodenum

E The tumour in contact with 75% of the superior mesenteric artery

Answer on page 200

QUESTION 42

An 82-year-old woman is referred to the on-call surgical team as an emergency admission. The patient lives in a residential care home and has a 48-hour history of generalised abdominal pain and vomiting. On examination, she is dehydrated and tachycardic and an abdominal radiograph demonstrates multiple dilated small bowel loops measuring up to 4.8 cm in diameter. A linear gas-filled structure is present in the right upper quadrant with short branches extending from it. What is the most likely diagnosis?

A Acute mesenteric ischaemia

B Emphysematous cholecystitis

C Gallstone ileus

D Obstructed right inguinal hernia

E Small bowel obstruction due to adhesions

Answer on page 200

QUESTION 43

A 72-year-old man presents with a 3-month history of significant weight loss, upper abdominal pain and pruritus. On examination the patient is clinically jaundiced and cachectic. A contrast-enhanced CT of the abdomen demonstrates marked intrahepatic biliary dilatation, a dilated common bile duct and a mass in the pancreatic head. An attempted ERCP fails as the ampulla of Vater cannot be cannulated. The patient attends the Radiology Department for percutaneous biliary drainage. Which one of the following statements is true?

A Biliary sepsis is an absolute contraindication to percutaneous biliary drainage.

B Excessive contrast injection into the intrahepatic ducts is a recognised cause of septic shock.

C If a malignant stricture is potentially resectable, a metallic biliary stent should be inserted.

D Percutaneous transhepatic cholangiography (PTC) is performed under general anaesthesia in the majority of cases.

E Prophylactic antibiotics are not routinely used in PTC.

Answer on page 200

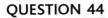

QUESTION 44

A 47-year-old man is knocked off his motorcycle and brought to the Emergency Department. On examination, he is haemodynamically stable but has left upper quadrant tenderness. A contrast-enhanced CT of the abdomen is performed and shows no evidence of visceral injury. The reporting radiologist notices a solitary, well-defined lesion in the large bowel that is of lower attenuation than the surrounding colonic wall. Which single additional finding would be most consistent with a colonic lipoma?

A There is a mean density of −10 HU on CT.

B Mucosal ulceration is seen on colonoscopy.

C On ultrasound, the lesion changes shape when compressed.

D The lesion lies in the sigmoid colon.

E There is a one-month history of rectal bleeding and weight loss.

Answer on page 201

QUESTION 45

A 31-year-old woman has a 6-month history of intermittent right upper quadrant pain. An abdominal ultrasound examination is performed and reveals a 3-cm hyperechoic mass in segment 6 of the liver. She undergoes an MRI examination of the liver with intravenous gadolinium. On the precontrast T1w images, the signal intensity of the lesion is isointense to surrounding liver parenchyma. Which one of the following statements is true regarding the post-gadolinium T1w images?

A Focal fatty infiltration demonstrates enhancement in the arterial phase.

B HCC usually enhance in the delayed phase images only.

C Hepatic adenomas typically demonstrate uniform enhancement in the arterial phase.

D Hypervascular metastases are typically hyperintense on T1 precontrast.

E Progressive centripetal enhancement in the portal venous and delayed phases is seen with HCC.

Answer on page 201

QUESTION 46

A 32-year-old man attends the Emergency Department 2 hours after he was assaulted outside a night club. On examination, he is haemodynamically stable with abrasions and tenderness over the lower left chest. The patient reports that he sustained significant abdominal injuries following an assault 7 years ago. A contrast-enhanced CT of the chest and abdomen is performed and demonstrates a fracture of the left 10th rib, but no intrathoracic injury. There is no visible spleen but multiple small nodules of uniformly enhancing soft tissue are present in the left upper quadrant and extend to the left iliac fossa. No peritoneal free fluid is demonstrated. What is the most likely diagnosis?

A Asplenia

B Polysplenia

C Shattered spleen

D Splenosis

E Wandering spleen

Answer on page 201

QUESTION 47

A 52-year-old man has a 3-year history of dysphagia and heartburn. There is no history of haematemesis and the patient's weight is stable. A barium swallow is performed and demonstrates a smooth narrowing of the mid-oesophagus. Small, saccular projections of barium are seen at the level of the stricture, extending perpendicular to the oesophagus. What is the cause of this appearance?

A Aphthous ulceration

B *Candida albicans* plaques

C Epiphrenic pulsion diverticulae

D Infiltration by adjacent non small cell lung cancer

E Intramural pseudodiverticulosis

Answer on page 201

QUESTION 48

A 42-year-old man has a history of alcohol excess and a previous duodenal ulcer. He presents to the Emergency Department with a 1-day history of epigastric pain and vomiting. Initial laboratory investigations are remarkable for a grossly elevated serum amylase and the patient is treated with intravenous fluids and analgesia. Six days later, his condition deteriorates and he develops a temperature of 39°C. A contrast-enhanced CT of the pancreas is performed. Which one of the following findings would be most indicative of infected pancreatic necrosis?

A An area of nonenhancement in the pancreatic body containing a locule of gas

B Diffuse enlargement of the pancreas with peripancreatic fat stranding

C Focal enlargement of the pancreatic head with reduced enhancement

D Splenic artery pseudoaneurysm formation adjacent to the pancreatic tail

E Splenic vein thrombosis extending to the superior mesenteric vein

Answer on page 202

QUESTION 49

A 27-year-old woman is referred to the gastroenterology outpatient clinic with a 3-month history of upper abdominal pain. There is no past medical history of note, but her sister has recently been diagnosed with a 'brain tumour'. A contrast-enhanced CT (portal venous phase) of the abdomen demonstrates a multicystic lesion in the head of the pancreas. The lesion contains 10 cysts measuring up to 15 mm in size with a small amount of calcification centrally. Several larger cysts are present in the pancreatic body and tail and both kidneys contain cortical cysts. What is the most likely underlying diagnosis?

A Autosomal dominant polycystic kidney disease

B Cystic fibrosis

C HHT

D Tuberous sclerosis

E Von Hippel Lindau disease (VHL)

Answer on page 202

QUESTION 50

A 38-year-old woman presents to her GP with a 3-month history of lethargy, nausea and itching. She was diagnosed with ulcerative colitis 8 years ago and has been treated with short courses of steroids and long-term oral mesalazine. Blood tests demonstrate an elevated serum bilirubin with markedly high alkaline phosphatase. MRCP demonstrates multiple biliary strictures with small diverticulae arising from the common duct. Which statement is true regarding the underlying diagnosis?

A Ten to 20% of patients have inflammatory bowel disease.

B Cessation of anti-inflammatory medication leads to normalisation of the liver function tests.

C It is also known as the type 5 choledochal cyst.

D Only the extrahepatic biliary ducts are involved.

E There is a significant increased risk of cholangiocarcinoma.

Answer on page 202

QUESTION 51

A 66-year-old man undergoes screening for colorectal cancer and is found to have two positive stool samples for faecal occult blood. The patient is asymptomatic with no significant medical history. He is referred for CT colonography (CTC). Which one of the following statements is correct regarding CTC?

A As much as 0.5–1% of examinations result in colonic perforation.

B A routine examination should involve supine imaging only.

C Significant extracolonic pathology is identified in 30–40% of symptomatic patients.

D The administration of intravenous contrast (portal venous imaging) is advised for asymptomatic patients, as it improves the detection of colonic neoplasms.

E The use of an antispasmodic (eg Buscopan) immediately prior to gas insufflation enables optimal colonic distension.

Answer on page 202

QUESTION 52

A 71-year-old woman is referred to the on-call surgical team as an emergency admission. She complains of a 1-week history of lower abdominal pain, nausea and vomiting. She has passed loose bowel motions over the past 2 days with no bleeding per rectum. She experienced a similar, less severe, episode of lower abdominal pain 2 years ago that resolved spontaneously.
On examination, the patient is pyrexial and tender in the left iliac fossa. Blood tests reveal elevated inflammatory markers and white cell count.
What would be the most likely findings on a contrast-enhanced CT?

A A thickened segment of sigmoid colon with mesenteric stranding and a small pericolonic fluid collection

B Annular thickening of the sigmoid colon with several enlarged local lymph nodes

C Areas of wall thickening throughout the colon with fistulous tracts between bowel loops

D Extensive pneumoperitoneum

E Extensive wall thickening of the rectum, sigmoid and descending colon with minimal pericolonic stranding

Answer on page 203

QUESTION 53

An 80-year-old man is referred to the gastroenterology outpatient clinic with a
1-year history of dysphagia. He describes worsening difficulty swallowing
solids and liquids with associated loss of 3 kg in weight. The past medical
history includes Parkinson's disease and right lower lobe pneumonia 6 months
ago. An upper gastrointestinal endoscopy is normal and the patient is
referred for a contrast swallow examination for suspected oesophageal
dysmotility. Which statement is true regarding this examination?

A If aspiration is suspected, water-soluble meglumine diatrizoate (Gastrografin) should be used initially.

B In suspected oesophageal dysmotility, an antispasmodic (eg Buscopan)
should be administered prior to prone swallow.

C Motility of the mid- and lower oesophagus is best assessed with the
patient standing erect in the left anterior oblique position.

D Repeated swallowing should be avoided and only single boluses of barium be used to assess for oesophageal dysmotility.

E Secondary oesophageal contractions are chaotic and do not propel the
barium bolus.

Answer on page 203

QUESTION 54

A 72-year-old man is referred to hospital as an emergency admission by his GP. He has experienced vomiting and abdominal pain for 24 hours following a takeaway meal. There is a past medical history of ischaemic heart disease, chronic obstructive pulmonary disease and hypertension. An abdominal radiograph is performed and demonstrates several gas-filled loops of small bowel centrally measuring up to 2.5 cm diameter. In the left side of the abdomen, multiple round foci of gas are projected over the wall of a loop of large bowel. No free gas or mucosal thickening is identified. What is the most likely explanation for the clinical and radiographic findings?

A Gastroenteritis with incidental pneumatosis coli

B Emphysematous pyelonephritis with a paralytic ileus

C Ischaemic colitis causing intramural bowel gas

D Perforated sigmoid diverticulitis with gas in the retroperitoneum

E Small bowel obstruction due to a gallstone ileus

Answer on page 203

QUESTION 55

A 68-year-old woman presents with a 2-month history of generalised abdominal bloating and two episodes of vaginal bleeding. On examination, the abdomen is distended with clinical evidence of ascites. Tumour markers are performed; CA 15-3 is normal, CA 125 and CEA are slightly elevated and CA 19-9 is markedly elevated. An abdominopelvic ultrasound demonstrates a moderate volume of ascites, multiple liver metastases and bilateral mixed solid/cystic adnexal masses. What is the most likely underlying primary tumour?

A Breast cancer

B Gastric adenocarcinoma

C Melanoma

D Ovarian cancer

E Primary peritoneal carcinoma

Answer on page 203

QUESTION 56

A 30-year-old male patient arrives at the Radiology Department for a barium follow-through examination. He has experienced chronic lower abdominal pain with weight loss and intermittent diarrhoea. Optical colonoscopy was normal. As the Specialist Registrar in the department, it is your responsibility to supervise this investigation and the radiographer asks how you would like the examination performed. Which statement is true regarding the barium follow-through examination?

A A 250% weight-to-volume barium sulphate should be used.

B Barium reaches the caecum within 30 minutes in the majority of patients.

C Barium sulphate suspensions are nonionic to avoid clumping of particles.

D Oral metoclopramide may be used to delay gastric emptying.

E The first radiograph should be a supine film after 60 minutes.

Answer on page 204

QUESTION 57

A 53-year-old man is seen in the liver transplant outpatient clinic. Two years ago, he underwent an orthotopic liver transplant for alcoholic liver disease and currently takes oral cyclosporin. He reports a 3-month history of weight loss and his liver function tests are found to be abnormal. A contrast-enhanced CT demonstrates multiple new low attenuation lesions within the liver. There is also marked thickening of several small bowel loops. What is the most likely diagnosis?

A Chronic graft ischaemia with portal hypertension

B Cyclosporin hepatotoxicity

C Multifocal hepatocellular carcinoma

D Post transplant lymphoproliferative disorder (PTLD)

E Secondary amyloidosis

Answer on page 204

QUESTION 58

A 29-year-old woman received a living related bone marrow transplant for chronic myeloid leukaemia 13 days ago. She has experienced bloody diarrhoea and severe lower abdominal pain for the past 4 days and an abdominal radiograph demonstrates prominent loops of gas-filled large bowel. A contrast-enhanced CT of the abdomen is performed and shows moderate wall thickening of the right hemicolon and terminal ileum with mesenteric fat stranding. There is no abdominal lymphadenopathy and the rectum and sigmoid colon appear normal. What is the most likely diagnosis?

A Crohn's disease
B Cytomegalovirus (CMV) colitis
C Neutropenic colitis
D PTLD
E Pseudomembranous colitis

Answer on page 204

QUESTION 59

A 33-year-old man presents to his GP with a 6-month history of increasing epigastric pain and vomiting. An upper GI endoscopy demonstrates multiple small ulcers in the gastric antrum and first and second parts of the duodenum. Biopsies show benign ulceration and are negative for *Helicobacter pylori*. The patient's symptoms do not improve on a high-dose oral proton pump inhibitor and an abdominal ultrasound demonstrates a well-defined 2-cm hypoechoic lesion in the pancreatic head. Which statement is true regarding the most likely underlying diagnosis?

A Ten to 20% of the pancreatic lesions are malignant.
B The condition is part of the type 2 multiple endocrine neoplasia syndrome.
C The pancreatic lesion is solitary in 80–90% of cases.
D The pancreatic lesion will enhance avidly on contrast-enhanced CT.
E There will be flattening of duodenal folds on a double contrast barium meal.

Answer on page 204

QUESTION 60

A 32-year-old man with Crohn's disease reports increased perianal pain and swelling over a 2-month period. On examination, there is a small perineal sinus lying at the 3 o'clock position in relation to the anus. On MRI, a fistulous track of high T2 signal is seen to pass from the anal canal, through the internal sphincter and then runs medial to the external sphincter. The track reaches the skin surface of the perineum and correlates with the sinus opening on physical examination. Which description best describes this anal fistula?

A Extrasphincteric

B Infrasphincteric

C Intersphincteric

D Suprasphincteric

E Trans-sphincteric

Answer on page 205

QUESTION 61

A 32-year-old woman undergoes a laparoscopic cholecystectomy for gallstones. Seven days later, she presents to the Emergency Department with increasing abdominal pain and fevers. On examination, her temperature is 39.6°C, HR = 100 bpm and BP = 110/60 mmHg with tenderness and guarding in the right upper and lower quadrants of the abdomen. Laboratory investigations reveal a grossly elevated CRP level and white cell count. The clinical team request a contrast-enhanced CT for suspected intra-abdominal sepsis. Which statement is true regarding intra-abdominal fluid collections?

A Fluid in the lesser sac communicates freely with the left subphrenic space.

B Fluid in the right paracolic gutter communicates freely into the pelvis and superiorly to the right subdiaphragmatic space.

C Fluid in the right paracolic gutter will be bounded superiorly by the phrenicocolic ligament.

D Postoperative gallbladder collections usually lie in the right infracolic space.

E The right subphrenic space is also called 'Morrison's pouch'.

Answer on page 205

QUESTION 62

A 79-year-old man is brought to the Emergency Department with generalised abdominal pain and vomiting for 5 days. He has not opened his bowels or passed flatus during this period and has been immobile for the past 48 hours. On examination, he is dehydrated with a distended abdomen and increased bowel sounds. An abdominal radiograph is performed and shows dilated loops of large bowel, measuring up to 5 cm in diameter. Dilated small bowel is present centrally but there is no evidence of perforation. Which statement is true regarding this clinical setting?

A Colonic pseudo-obstruction is a recognised cause of these radiographic findings.

B Diverticulitis is the most common cause of large bowel obstruction in the UK.

C Obstruction of the large bowel occurs more commonly on the right side of the colon than the left.

D Paralytic ileus is excluded by these radiographic findings.

E The ileocaecal valve is not competent in this patient.

Answer on page 205

QUESTION 63

A 17-year-old man has a 2-month history of abdominal pain and rectal bleeding. Clinical examination is unremarkable and a flexible sigmoidoscopy is normal. A Tc-99 m pertechnetate study is performed, demonstrating abnormal activity in the lower abdomen. One month later, the patient presents to the Emergency Department with acute abdominal pain and vomiting. A contrast-enhanced CT of the abdomen shows an ileocolic intussusception. What is the most likely underlying diagnosis?

A Colonic lipoma

B Crohn's disease

C Meckel's diverticulum

D Small bowel adenocarcinoma

E Whipple's disease

Answer on page 206

QUESTION 64

A 27-year-old man is referred to the hepatology outpatient clinic with a 3-week history of malaise, lethargy and mild upper abdominal pain. Liver function tests performed by his GP are significantly abnormal. The results of hepatitis serology performed in the clinic are consistent with an acute hepatitis B infection. An abdominal ultrasound is performed. What is the most likely finding on ultrasound?

A Decreased reflectivity of the liver parenchyma

B Increased reflectivity of the liver parenchyma

C Nodular liver surface

D Normal ultrasound appearances

E Retrograde portal venous flow

Answer on page 206

QUESTION 65

A 49-year-old woman is an emergency admission to the surgical admissions unit with a 5-day history of upper abdominal pain. On clinical examination, there is right upper quadrant tenderness and laboratory investigations show an elevated white cell count and CRP. An abdominal ultrasound is performed, but is of limited value due to the patient's body habitus and the gallbladder is poorly visualised. The patient undergoes dynamic radioisotope hepatobiliary scintigraphy with an intravenous injection of a Tc-99 m-labelled pharmaceutical. Which one of the following statements is true regarding radioisotope hepatobiliary scintigraphy?

A Increased isotope activity in the region of the gallbladder is consistent with acute cholecystitis.

B Nonvisualisation of the gallbladder after 2 hours is consistent with acute cholecystitis.

C Sulphur colloid is the most commonly used pharmaceutical in this examination.

D The administration of intravenous morphine causes sphincter of Oddi relaxation.

E Visualisation of isotope activity in the duodenum is abnormal.

Answer on page 206

QUESTION 66

A 79-year-old woman trips and falls whilst stepping off a bus. She suffers a fractured right neck of femur and undergoes a hemiarthroplasty the following day. Her early recovery is complicated by bronchopneumonia which resolves after 5 days of broad spectrum antibiotics. On her tenth day in hospital she develops abdominal pain and diarrhoea and pseudomembranous colitis is suspected clinically. Which one of the following statements is true regarding pseudomembranous colitis?

A A normal abdominal CT effectively excludes pseudomembranous colitis.

B Ascites is present in up to 40% of patients.

C CT carries a low positive predictive value for pseudomembranous colitis.

D Extensive pericolonic stranding is a typical feature on CT.

E The rectum is not involved in 40–50% of patients.

Answer on page 206

QUESTION 67

A 63-year-old man attends the Radiology Department for an MRCP. He was recently found to have abnormal liver function tests and an abdominal ultrasound showed multiple stones in the gallbladder with a dilated common bile duct. The surgical team have requested the MRCP to assess whether there are gallstones in the bile ducts. Which statement is true regarding MRCP in this setting?

A Blood in the biliary tree is a recognised cause of a false positive MRCP.

B MRCP diagnostic quality reduces as the serum bilirubin rises.

C MRCP is reliant on contrast excretion into the biliary tree.

D The sensitivity of MRCP for choledocholithiasis is 60–70%.

E The sequences are heavily T1 weighted in the majority of cases.

Answer on page 207

QUESTION 68

A 45-year-old man undergoes an upper GI endoscopy following a 2-month history of weight loss and dysphagia to solids. The endoscopy demonstrates a tumour in the mid-oesophagus and biopsies confirm a squamous cell carcinoma. An endoscopic ultrasound is subsequently performed and demonstrates a hypoechoic tumour mass in the anterior aspect of the mid-oesophagus. The tumour is seen to infiltrate the muscularis propria and extends beyond the serosal surface of the oesophagus. Which structure is most at risk of direct invasion by this oesophageal tumour?

A Azygos vein

B Left lobe of liver

C Left main bronchus

D Right diaphragmatic crus

E Right ventricle

Answer on page 207

QUESTION 69

A 51-year-old man attends the Emergency Department with a 3-hour history of sudden onset lower abdominal pain and vomiting. On examination, there is tenderness in the right iliac fossa but laboratory investigations are remarkable only for a mildly elevated CRP level. A contrast-enhanced CT of the abdomen is performed and demonstrates an ovoid mass lying medial to the caecum with high attenuation stranding in the pericolic fat and a central area of low density (−150 HU). There is no colonic wall thickening identified. What is the diagnosis?

A Acute appendicitis

B Epiploic appendagitis

C Ileocaecal tuberculosis

D Meckel's diverticulum

E Right-sided diverticulitis

Answer on page 207

QUESTION 70

A 67-year-old man is referred to the gastroenterology outpatient clinic with a 6-week history of upper abdominal pain, vomiting and weight loss. The patient has previously been fit and well but has lost 10 kg in weight during this period. Clinical examination and laboratory investigations are unremarkable. A contrast-enhanced CT of the abdomen is performed and demonstrates extensive thickening of the gastric body and antrum. Which additional feature would make a diagnosis of gastric carcinoma more likely than gastric lymphoma?

A Direct invasion of the left lobe of liver

B Coeliac axis lymphadenopathy

C Preserved perigastric fat planes

D Previous *Helicobacter pylori* infection

E Regional lymphadenopathy

Answer on page 207

QUESTION 71

A 62-year-old woman presents to the Emergency Department with a 2-day history of excruciating abdominal pain and is found to have an elevated serum amylase. An abdominal ultrasound demonstrates multiple stones in the gallbladder but there is no biliary dilatation and the pancreas is obscured by bowel gas. The patient's clinical condition deteriorates and a contrast-enhanced CT is performed. This demonstrates ill-defined enlargement of the pancreas with infiltration of the peripancreatic fat. The peripancreatic fluid is localised only to the anterior pararenal space. Which one other structure also lies in the anterior pararenal space?

A Descending colon

B Gallbladder

C Kidneys

D Spleen

E Stomach

Answer on page 207

QUESTION 72

A 35-year-old man has a history of excess alcohol intake and is referred for an abdominal ultrasound by his GP. This demonstrates a 3-cm area of increased reflectivity within liver segment 4a. The lesion does not have any mass effect on adjacent vessels and has a geographic margin. A diagnosis of focal fat deposition is suspected and an MRI of the liver is performed. Which MRI artefact can be utilised to confirm this diagnosis?

A Aliasing

B Chemical shift

C Magic angle

D Susceptibility

E Truncation

Answer on page 208

QUESTION 73

A 40-year-old woman has a 15-year history of ulcerative colitis (UC). After the initial diagnosis, she suffered frequent exacerbations of colitis requiring several hospital admissions. She declined surgical intervention at that stage and has subsequently been well controlled on medical management. Recently, she has developed a change in bowel habit and a double contrast barium enema is performed. This shows a stricture in the descending colon. Which one statement is true regarding strictures in ulcerative colitis?

A Abrupt shouldering is typical of a benign stricture in UC.

B In patients with UC, colorectal carcinomas typically arise from tubular adenomas.

C The majority of strictures in UC are benign.

D There is no increased risk of colorectal carcinoma in patients with UC.

E Widening of the presacral space is pathognomonic of a rectal carcinoma.

Answer on page 208

QUESTION 74

A 17-year-old man is referred to the gastroenterology outpatient clinic with iron deficiency anaemia. The patient is otherwise well with no gastrointestinal symptoms and a normal physical examination. Endoscopic examination of the upper and lower gastrointestinal tract is normal. A mesenteric catheter angiogram is performed and demonstrates a persistent vitelline artery. What is the diagnosis?

A Behçet's disease

B Colonic arteriovenous malformation

C Intestinal lymphangiectasia

D Meckel's diverticulum

E Small bowel angiodysplasia

Answer on page 208

QUESTION 75

An 81-year-old man presents with a 3-month history of weight loss and upper abdominal pain. Serum amylase is normal but CA 19-9 is elevated and liver function tests are abnormal. An abdominal ultrasound demonstrates mild intrahepatic biliary dilatation with common bile duct measuring 16 mm in diameter. The pancreatic head is obscured by bowel gas and a contrast-enhanced CT of the abdomen is performed. What is the most likely finding in the pancreas?

A A 1-cm intensely enhancing mass in the pancreatic body

B A 6-cm septated cyst in the pancreatic tail

C Diffusely enlarged pancreas with peripancreatic fluid collection

D Hypovascular mass in the pancreatic head

E Pancreatic ductal calcification and atrophy

Answer on page 208

QUESTION 76

A 74-year-old man attends the Radiology Department for an abdominal ultrasound examination. He has a 2-month history of nausea and vomiting with unexplained weight loss. On ultrasound, there are linear structures of high reflectivity seen within liver segments 2–4. On turning into the left lateral decubitus position, similar hyperechoic structures become visible in the right lobe of liver. What additional medical history would explain these findings?

A Autosomal dominant polycystic kidney disease

B ERCP and sphincterotomy

C Previous *Pneumocystis jiroveci (carinii)* infection

D Right hemicolectomy for colorectal cancer

E Wilson's disease

Answer on page 209

QUESTION 77

A 48-year-old man has a strong family history of colorectal cancer. He is found to have a mild microcytic anaemia and a stool sample for faecal occult blood testing is positive. A CT colonography is performed and, on 3D images, a 1-cm focal polypoid mass is seen in the wall of the sigmoid colon. The reporting radiologist is unsure whether this lesion is significant and reviews the 2D supine and prone axial images. Which additional feature would be most consistent with a polyp?

A The lesion contains a locule of gas at its base.

B The lesion has a mean density of -150 HU.

C The lesion is of homogeneous attenuation.

D The lesion lies on the dependent surface of the bowel on prone and supine images.

E There are diverticulae seen in the sigmoid colon.

Answer on page 209

QUESTION 78

A 23-year-old man presents with a 2-day history of vomiting and generalised abdominal pain. Two years ago, he underwent a small bowel resection for an ileal stricture due to Crohn's disease. Initial blood tests reveal a raised CRP and white cell count and an abdominal radiograph demonstrates dilated loops of small bowel. Small bowel obstruction is suspected and a contrast-enhanced CT of the abdomen is performed. Which one of the following statements is true regarding the role of multidetector CT in small bowel obstruction?

A Five to 15% of small bowel obstructions are due to hernias.

B Twenty to 30% of small bowel obstructions are due to adhesions.

C Bowel wall thickening and intramural gas indicate the presence of pneumatosis coli.

D Closed loop obstruction is less likely to result in bowel ischaemia than simple obstruction.

E In small bowel obstruction due to adhesions, a transition point will not be seen.

Answer on page 209

QUESTION 79

A 27-year-old woman is admitted to hospital with an episode of mild acute pancreatitis. An abdominal ultrasound demonstrates no gallstones or biliary dilatation and the pancreas appears normal. She is managed conservatively and discharged after 7 days. Three months later, she is seen in the outpatient clinic and complains of worsening upper abdominal pain. A contrast-enhanced CT demonstrates a 6-cm cystic mass in the pancreatic body with a thin enhancing wall. Which statement is true regarding this cystic pancreatic mass?

A Forty to 60% will resolve spontaneously.

B Eighty to 90% occur within 7 days of acute pancreatitis.

C Gas within the lesion would be pathognomonic of an enteric fistula.

D Surgical drainage will be required to confirm the diagnosis.

E The cyst fluid is likely to have low amylase content.

Answer on page 209

QUESTION 80

A 67-year-old woman undergoes surgical resection of a distal sigmoid adenocarcinoma. The surgeon performs a primary anastomosis between the descending colon and rectum and leaves a defunctioning loop colostomy. Nine days later, the patient is experiencing fevers and low abdominal pain. A contrast-enhanced CT shows a small fluid collection around the anastomosis with no definite abscess identified. The surgical team are concerned about the integrity of the anastomosis. Which investigation would you choose to look for an anastomotic leak?

A Barium enema

B Barium follow-through

C MRI pelvis with intravenous gadolinium

D Water-soluble contrast cystogram

E Water-soluble contrast enema

Answer on page 210

QUESTION 81

A 64-year-old woman presents to her GP with increasing discomfort in her upper abdomen and anorexia. There is a past medical history of gallstones. The GP requests an abdominal ultrasound and this demonstrates a 6 × 4 cm mixed echogenicity lesion in the gallbladder fossa, with the gallbladder not separately visualised. On CT, the gallbladder fossa mass demonstrates central low attenuation with peripheral enhancement and mild intrahepatic biliary dilatation. Low attenuation lymph nodes are present at the porta hepatis (measuring up to 1.5 cm short axis). Which diagnosis is most likely?

A Adenomyomatosis

B Gallbladder carcinoma

C Hepatocellular carcinoma

D Porcelain gallbladder

E Xanthogranulomatous cholecystitis

Answer on page 210

QUESTION 82

A 52-year-old man is investigated for weight loss and dyspepsia. At endoscopy, an adenocarcinoma of the posterior wall of the gastric body is visualised and confirmed on histology. A contrast-enhanced CT of the abdomen is performed (with intravenous Buscopan and water as oral contrast) to stage the tumour. The primary tumour is seen as focal gastric mucosal thickening with a small amount of free fluid noted in the left paracolic gutter and pelvis. An endoscopic ultrasound is performed and shows that the tumour extends beyond the serosal surface of the posterior gastric wall. Which structure is most at risk of direct invasion by this tumour?

A Abdominal aorta
B Left lobe of liver
C Pancreas
D Right diaphragmatic crus
E Transverse colon

Answer on page 210

QUESTION 83

A 22-year-old woman attends the Emergency Department with a 10-day history of vomiting and diarrhoea. The symptoms have worsened and are now associated with severe abdominal pain. Initial investigations reveal an elevated neutrophil count and CRP and she is treated with intravenous fluids and antiemetics. In view of increased pain and fever, a contrast-enhanced CT of the abdomen and pelvis is performed and shows that a segment of bowel is significantly thickened. The microbiology laboratory telephones the clinical team and states that *Yersinia enterocolitica* has been isolated from the patient's stool samples. Which segment of the bowel is likely to be abnormal?

A Duodenum
B Gastric antrum
C Proximal jejenum
D Sigmoid colon
E Terminal ileum

Answer on page 210

QUESTION 84

A 74-year-old woman is referred to hospital by her GP as an emergency medical admission. The referral letter indicates that the patient is in residential care and has Alzheimer's disease. Her carers have noticed generalised malaise and significant weight loss over the past 6 weeks. A contrast-enhanced CT is performed and demonstrates multiple low attenuation liver metastases. These lesions contain foci of amorphous calcification and show rim enhancement in the portal venous phase. What is the most likely underlying malignancy in this patient?

A Carcinoid tumour of ileum
B Endometrial carcinoma
C Mucinous adenocarcinoma of colon
D Multifocal hepatocellular carcinoma
E Papillary carcinoma of thyroid

Answer on page 210

QUESTION 85

A 79-year-old woman is admitted to hospital with a 2-day history of diarrhoea and abdominal pain. A contrast-enhanced CT of the abdomen demonstrates mucosal thickening of the proximal descending colon with a low attenuation 'target sign' appearance. The rectosigmoid and right hemicolon are normal in appearance. The patient is managed conservatively and the symptoms resolve. Six months later, a double contrast barium enema is performed and shows an irregular stricture of the descending colon with barium sacculation. What was the original diagnosis?

A Acute diverticulitis
B Giardiasis
C Ischaemic colitis
D Pseudomembranous colitis
E Ulcerative colitis

Answer on page 211

QUESTION 86

A 32-year-old man presents to his GP with increasing pain on swallowing solids and liquids. He has lost 15 kg in weight over the preceding 2 months. After a full history and examination, he is found to be HIV positive with a very low CD4 count. The GP refers him for a barium swallow examination and this demonstrates a single ulcer in the mid-oesophagus. The ulcer has a smooth margin, measures 4 cm in length and is oval in shape. There is no stricture identified. Which diagnosis is most likely?

A Candida oesophagitis

B CMV oesophagitis

C Intramural pseudodiverticulosis

D Oesophageal lymphoma

E Squamous cell carcinoma of the oesophagus

Answer on page 211

QUESTION 87

A 46-year-old woman was diagnosed with breast cancer 3 months ago. A recent abdominal ultrasound identified a solitary liver lesion and an MRI of the liver is performed. This demonstrates a 2.5-cm diameter mass in liver segment 8. This lesion has a well-defined, lobulated contour and yields high T2 signal. An extended echo time of 180 ms is used and the lesion remains of high T2 signal (greater than the spleen, less than CSF). What is the most likely diagnosis?

A Breast cancer metastasis

B Focal nodular hyperplasia

C Haemangioma

D Hepatic adenoma

E Simple liver cyst

Answer on page 211

QUESTION 88

A 49-year-old woman has experienced increasing difficulty swallowing over the past 6 months, with associated retrosternal discomfort. A barium swallow is performed and demonstrates virtually no peristaltic activity within a dilated oesophagus. The gastro-oesophageal junction appears widened and there is marked reflux of barium when the patient lies supine. An upper GI endoscopy shows moderate reflux oesophagitis. Given these findings, what is the most likely underlying diagnosis?

A Achalasia

B Oesophageal web

C Presbyoesophagus

D Scleroderma

E Squamous cell carcinoma of oesophagus

Answer on page 211

QUESTION 89

A 44-year-old man has liver cirrhosis due to chronic hepatitis B infection. He is admitted to hospital with decompensated liver disease and a serum alpha fetoprotein level is found to be markedly elevated. An abdominal ultrasound demonstrates a 3-cm hypoechoic mass in liver segment 5 with no colour flow demonstrated in an adjacent branch of the portal vein. The ultrasound probe is positioned over this focal lesion and an intravenous microbubble contrast agent is injected in the patient's left arm. At what stage will this liver lesion appear most echogenic?

A Pre contrast injection

B 15–30 seconds post injection

C 60–80 seconds post injection

D 5 minutes post injection

E 10 minutes post injection

Answer on page 211

QUESTION 90

A 41-year-old man has a 3 month history of weight loss and recurrent central abdominal pain. The pain is intermittent and radiates from the epigastrium through to his back. His past medical history includes excessive alcohol consumption and two previous admissions to hospital for acute pancreatitis. A contrast-enhanced CT of the abdomen is performed with precontrast, arterial and portal venous phase images of the upper abdomen. Which CT finding would be more suggestive of chronic pancreatitis than ductal pancreatic adenocarcinoma?

A Common bile duct dilatation
B Focal enlargement of the pancreatic head
C Intraductal pancreatic calcification
D Peripancreatic fat stranding and ascites
E Reduced enhancement of body of pancreas

Answer on page 212

QUESTION 91

A 27-year-old woman presents to the Emergency Department with a 3-day history of sharp pain in the left iliac fossa. A transvaginal pelvic ultrasound is performed and shows a 5-cm unilocular cyst in the left ovary. The radiologist then performs a transabdominal ultrasound to assess the kidneys. It is noted that the liver parenchyma extends significantly below the right costal margin and passes anterior to the right kidney. The liver texture appears uniformly normal. What is the most likely explanation for the appearance of the liver?

A Biliary hamartoma
B Fitz-Hugh-Curtis syndrome
C Focal fatty infiltration
D Focal nodular hyperplasia (FNH)
E Riedel's lobe

Answer on page 212

QUESTION 92

A 56-year-old woman is found to have a 2.5-cm renal cell carcinoma in the upper pole of the right kidney. A contrast-enhanced CT of the chest and abdomen is performed and shows no evidence of local lymphadenopathy or distant metastases. The reporting radiologist notes a 2-cm cystic lesion in the pancreatic body. When assessing this cystic pancreatic lesion, which one of the following statements is true?

A Eighty to 90% of symptomatic cystic lesions are pseudocysts.

B Ninety to 95% of serous cystadenomas (microcystadenomas) contain calcification.

C An asymptomatic solitary 8-mm simple cyst requires mandatory follow-up.

D In a mucinous cystadenoma (macrocystadenoma), multiple small cysts typically measure up to 20 mm each.

E The majority of mucinous cystadenomas occur in the pancreatic head.

Answer on page 212

QUESTION 93

A 64-year-old man sees his GP with a 2-month history of unexplained weight loss. He has experienced right upper quadrant discomfort and blood tests show an elevated bilirubin and gamma glutamyltransferase (GGT) with grossly elevated alkaline phosphatase. An abdominal ultrasound performed 6 months ago was normal with no evidence of gallstones. Which factor would not increase this patient's risk of cholangiocarcinoma?

A Caroli's disease

B *Clonorchis sinensis* infection

C Exposure to iohexol 15 years ago

D Primary sclerosing cholangitis

E Type 1 choledochal cyst

Answer on page 213

QUESTION 94

A 71-year-old woman has a contrast-enhanced CT of the abdomen and pelvis to investigate lower abdominal pain and reduced bowel habit. An abnormal mesenteric soft tissue mass is present and displaces adjacent loops of bowel. The mass has multiple linear strands that radiate out towards the adjacent bowel loops giving a 'stellate' appearance. Which term describes this CT appearance?

A Aneurysmal dilatation

B Desmoplastic reaction

C Omental cake

D Peritoneal seeding

E Sandwich encasement

Answer on page 213

QUESTION 95

A 24-year-old man is referred to the gastroenterology outpatient clinic. He describes intermittent bloody diarrhoea with abdominal pain and has lost 5 kg in weight over the past 6 months. His father and uncle both have inflammatory bowel disease. Routine laboratory investigations are remarkable for a moderately elevated CRP. A double contrast barium enema examination is performed. Which of the following findings would be more consistent with Crohn's disease than ulcerative colitis?

A Aphthous ulceration interspersed with areas of normal mucosa

B Fine granular appearance of the descending and sigmoid colon

C Isolated involvement of the rectum and sigmoid

D Shortening and narrowing of the entire colon with absence of haustral folds

E The presence of 'collar button' ulceration

Answer on page 213

QUESTION 96

A 30-year-old man attends the Emergency Department with a 2-day history of abdominal pain and vomiting. On examination, he is afebrile with a firm mass palpable in the right lower quadrant of the abdomen. A supine abdominal radiograph is performed and demonstrates dilated loops of small bowel with a large soft tissue mass in the right lower quadrant. On ultrasound, the mass has a 'pseudotumour' appearance. What is the most likely diagnosis?

A Colonic carcinoma

B Gallstone ileus

C Intussusception

D Psoas abscess

E Strangulated femoral hernia

Answer on page 213

QUESTION 97

An 83-year-old man undergoes an emergency left hip hemiarthroplasty following a fractured neck of femur. Six days after surgery, he develops increasing abdominal distension with nausea and vomiting. An abdominal radiograph is performed and demonstrates dilatation of the ascending and transverse colon with the caecum measuring 7.0 cm in diameter. The clinical team believe that the patient may have colonic pseudo-obstruction and a single contrast (instant) enema is performed using water-soluble contrast. What are the likely findings in colonic pseudo-obstruction?

A Extrinsic compression of the sigmoid colon

B Long, irregular stricture of the sigmoid colon

C Long, smooth stricture at the splenic flexure

D No stricture demonstrated

E Short 'apple core' stricture of the descending colon

Answer on page 214

QUESTION 98

A 49-year-old man is involved in a road traffic accident and sustains serious head and chest injuries. He is ventilated on the intensive care unit and his injuries are managed conservatively. Ten days later, he develops a temperature of 39.5°, becomes tachycardic and requires inotropic support to maintain his blood pressure. An abdominal ultrasound is performed and shows a cystic structure in the right upper quadrant measuring 12 × 8 cm in size. The mass has a 6-mm thick wall, contains a layer of echogenic material and is surrounded by a rim of fluid. What is the most likely diagnosis?

A Acalculous cholecystitis

B Acute cholangitis

C Gallbladder haematoma

D Traumatic hepatic artery pseudoaneurysm

E Xanthogranulomatous cholecystitis

Answer on page 214

QUESTION 99

A 59-year-old woman is found to have several small lesions within the liver on abdominal ultrasound. The ultrasound had been requested for investigation of abnormal liver function tests. An MRI of the liver demonstrates several low T2 signal lesions within the liver parenchyma. These lesions yield high signal on T1w images and, following intravenous gadolinium, there is avid enhancement in the hepatic arterial phase. Which diagnosis would best explain these findings?

A Colorectal metastases

B Focal fatty infiltration

C Focal fatty sparing

D Melanoma metastases

E Multifocal HCC

Answer on page 214

QUESTION 100

A 72-year-old woman is brought to the Emergency Department with an 8-hour history of profuse fresh rectal bleeding. She had been awaiting endoscopic investigation of iron deficiency anaemia, but has no other significant medical history. On examination, she is haemodynamically unstable and blood tests reveal Hb = 5.0 g/dL. Following resuscitation, the patient's condition stabilises and the surgical team request radiological investigation to identify the source of GI bleeding. Which statement is true regarding this clinical scenario?

A Catheter angiography of the mesenteric vessels is the most sensitive method for detecting lower GI bleeding.

B Colorectal cancer is the most common cause of profuse lower GI haemorrhage.

C In fresh rectal bleeding, selective catheterisation of the coeliac axis is not required during catheter angiography.

D Isotope studies with Tc-99 m-labelled red blood cells can detect bleeding rates as low as 0.1 ml/min.

E The most common site of colonic angiodysplasia is the descending colon.

Answer on page 214

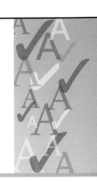

MODULE 3

Gastrointestinal

ANSWERS

QUESTION 1

ANSWER: C

Mucinous cystic pancreatic tumours (cystadenomas and cystadenocarcinomas) typically contain a few large cysts, each measuring more than 20 mm diameter.

Reference: *Grainger & Allison's* 5e, pp 804–806.

QUESTION 2

ANSWER: B

HCC derives its blood supply from the hepatic artery (hence the rapid arterial phase enhancement). A large HCC will usually demonstrate heterogeneous reflectivity due to areas of necrosis, but smaller lesions are typically of homogeneous low reflectivity on ultrasound. HCC often invades the branches of the portal vein and the most frequent site of metastases is the lungs. Metastases to the brain are typically hypervascular and do not usually contain calcification.

Reference: Yu SCH, Yeung DTK, So NMC. Imaging features of hepatocellular carcinoma *Clin Radiol* 2004;59:145–156.

QUESTION 3

ANSWER: E

A localised paralytic ileus due to inflammatory change in the pancreas is known as the sentinel loop sign.

Reference: *Grainger & Allison's* 5e, pp 598, 793–798.

QUESTION 4

ANSWER: C

Magenstrasse refers to the normal longitudinal mucosal folds seen adjacent to the lesser curve of the stomach during a barium meal. The 'bull's eye' appearance seen during a barium meal is due to a central ulcer in an elevated area of submucosa. A GIST may well have this appearance and neurofibromatosis can cause single or multiple target lesions. Melanoma is the commonest cause of submucosal gastric metastases.

Reference: Chapman S, Nakielny R. *Aids to Radiological Differential Diagnosis*, 5th edition (Edinburgh: Saunders, 2003), p 136.

QUESTION 5

ANSWER: D

Graded compression ultrasound of the appendix can avoid unnecessary surgery and ionising radiation—particularly relevant for children and women of childbearing age. The finding of a noncompressible appendix with transverse diameter of 6 mm or greater is highly suggestive of acute appendicitis (specificity 86–100%). Other ultrasound findings include hyperechoic fat in the right iliac fossa, periappendiceal fluid or a pelvic fluid collection (appendiceal abscess).

Reference: Gracey D, McClure MJ. The impact of ultrasound in suspected acute appendicitis. *Clin Radiol* 2007;62:573–578.

QUESTION 6

ANSWER: B

The presence of severe ulceration leading to mucosal islands is a major sign of toxic megacolon (the other key finding is colonic dilatation > 5 cm).

Reference: *Grainger & Allison's* 5e, p 696.

QUESTION 7

ANSWER: D

Following an ultrasound-guided liver biopsy, nearly two-thirds of complications occur in the first 2 hours, with 96% of complications having occurred by 24 hours.

Reference: *Grainger & Allison's* 5e, pp 758–759.

QUESTION 8

ANSWER: B

A significant minority of patients with hyperparathyroidism will develop acute pancreatitis and around 30% of these patients develop pancreatic calcification. Hypoparathyroidism is associated with calcification in the soft tissues but pancreatic calcification is not a recognised feature. Hereditary pancreatitis is an autosomal dominant condition with 60% of patients demonstrating round, coarse calcification of the pancreas.

Reference: Chapman & Nakielny, *Aids to Radiological Differential Diagnosis*, pp 181–182.

QUESTION 9

ANSWER: C

Focal fatty sparing usually leads to geographic or wedge-shaped lesions of reduced echogenicity. There should be no mass effect or abnormal enhancement characteristics in focal fatty sparing or infiltration. Both focal fatty sparing and infiltration typically occur in sites such as the gallbladder fossa, falciform ligament and porta hepatis, due to the altered venous drainage of these areas.

Reference: Karcaaltincaba M, Akhan O. Imaging of hepatic steatosis and fatty sparing. *Eur J Radiol* 2007;61:33–43.

QUESTION 10

ANSWER: A

Clinical features of oesophageal achalasia also include relief of retrosternal pain with carbonated and hot drinks (relaxes the lower oesophageal sphincter).

Reference: *Grainger & Allison's* 5e, p 621.

QUESTION 11

ANSWER: A

Most liver metastases are hypovascular and appear as lower attenuation than normal liver parenchyma on portal venous phase CT. Hypervascular metastases are less common and appear most prominently during the arterial phase (20–30 s) post contrast. Carcinoid, melanoma, thyroid and renal cancer are the most common causes of hypervascular liver metastases.

Reference: Chapman & Nakielny, *Aids to Radiological Differential Diagnosis*, pp 172–173.

QUESTION 12

ANSWER: C

The MRI findings are highly suggestive of a hepatic adenoma and the history of rapid growth during pregnancy is supportive of this diagnosis.

Reference: *Grainger & Allison's* 5e, pp 741–742.

QUESTION 13

ANSWER: C

The Couinaud classification divides the liver into 8 independent segments, each of which has its own vascular supply and biliary drainage. The portal vein separates the superior and inferior segments, with further division based on the relationship to the nearest hepatic veins. Because of this division into self-contained units, the Couinaud classification carries particular importance in the setting of resectable liver lesions, such as a solitary colorectal metastasis.

Reference: Chapman & Nakielny, *Aids to Radiological Differential Diagnosis*, p 166.

QUESTION 14

ANSWER: E

Evidence of peritoneal invasion indicates stage T4 rectal cancer.

Reference: *Grainger & Allison's* 5e, pp 689–690.

QUESTION 15

ANSWER: D

Hepatic artery thrombosis is the most common and serious early vascular complication post liver transplant. Thrombolysis is an option in this setting, but many patients will ultimately require retransplantation. Prompt and accurate diagnosis is therefore essential. A parvus et tardus waveform may be seen distal to stenosis of the hepatic artery, with associated elevated systolic velocity at the stenotic segment. Portal vein thrombosis is less common and can result in the acute development of ascites and varices. IVC thrombosis is rare and usually related to surgical technique, whilst an arterioportal fistula is an infrequent complication of liver biopsy.

Reference: Federle MP, Kapoor V. Complications of liver transplantation: imaging and intervention. *Radiol Clinics North Am* 2003;41(6):1289–1305.

QUESTION 16

ANSWER: B

A multiloculated cystic mass with daughter cysts and echogenic debris ('hydatid sand') is characteristic of a hydatid liver cyst.

Reference: *Grainger & Allison's* 5e, pp 736–737.

QUESTION 17

ANSWER: A

Cholesterol crystals within Rokitansky-Aschoff sinuses produce the characteristic 'comet tail' or ring-down artefact seen in adenomyomatosis. Both gallbladder carcinoma and adenomyomatosis can cause focal wall thickening in the gallbladder, but the visualisation of hyperechoic sinuses is typical of the latter. A porcelain gallbladder is a complication of chronic cholecystitis causing mural calcification: the gallbladder wall appears hyperechoic with marked acoustic shadowing.

Reference: Gore RM, Yaghmai V, Newmark GM, et al. Imaging benign and malignant disease of the gallbladder. *Radiol Clin North Am* 2002;40(6):1307–1323.

QUESTION 18

ANSWER: A

Hampton's line refers to a lucent line crossing the ulcer base: its presence is highly suggestive of a benign ulcer.

Reference: *Grainger & Allison's* 5e, pp 633–634.

QUESTION 19

ANSWER: B

Formation of a cystoduodenostomy drains the exocrine pancreatic secretions into a duodenal loop, anastomosed directly with the urinary bladder. Enteric drainage into small bowel can also be performed depending on surgical technique.

Reference: *Grainger & Allison's* 5e, p 807.

QUESTION 20

ANSWER: D

In oesophageal cancer, T1 tumours are limited to the mucosa only, T2 tumours invade the muscularis propria and T3 lesions extend into the adventitia. T4 lesions breach the serosal surface and can invade mediastinal structures.

Reference: *Grainger & Allison's* 5e, pp 616–619.

QUESTION 21

ANSWER: A

The presence of haustrations in a dilated viscus and gas in the appendix are key to the diagnosis of caecal volvulus.

Reference: *Grainger & Allison's* 5e, pp 597–598.

QUESTION 22

ANSWER: A

Brown fat is a well-recognised physiological cause of 18-FDG uptake (the location and symmetrical distribution are typical) and benzodiazepines can be administered to reduce brown fat uptake. Hyperglycaemia is likely to result in reduced 18-FDG uptake as the radioisotope has to compete with glucose for uptake into metabolically active cells.

Reference: El-Haddad G, Alavi A, Mavi A, et al. Normal variants in [18F]-fluorodeoxyglucose PET imaging. *Radiol Clin North Am* 2005;42(6):1063–1081.

QUESTION 23

ANSWER: A

This describes the characteristic 'hide bound' appearance of the small bowel in scleroderma.

Reference: *Grainger & Allison's* 5e, pp 668–675.

QUESTION 24

ANSWER: B

Autosomal dominant condition with multiple colonic adenomas and 100% risk of colorectal carcinoma 20 years after diagnosis. Associated with hamartomas in the stomach, gastric and duodenal adenomas and periampullary carcinoma.

References: *Grainger & Allison's* 5e, pp 683–685.
Chapman & Nakielny, *Aids to Radiological Differential Diagnosis*, pp 148–149.

QUESTION 25

ANSWER: D

In iron overload due to recurrent transfusions, there is increased iron deposition in the reticuloendothelial system. This leads to reduced T1, T2 and T2* signal intensity in the liver and spleen. Haemochromatosis causes diffusely reduced T2 signal in the liver and may lead to cirrhosis, but the splenic signal intensity should remain normal. Diffuse fatty liver will lead to increased T2 signal in the liver with signal loss during out-of-phase images.

Reference: Martin DR, Danrad R, Hussain SM. MR imaging of the liver. *Radiol Clin North Am* 2005;43(5):861–881.

QUESTION 26

ANSWER: D

It appears that relative stenosis of the cranially sited minor papilla results in increased risk of pancreatitis in these patients.

Reference: *Grainger & Allison's* 5e, pp 790–792.

QUESTION 27

ANSWER: A

Acute symptoms are not an accurate predictor of chronic radiation enteritis. The valvulae conniventes are typically thickened in acute radiation enteritis and the distal jejunum and ileum are the most frequent sites of small bowel involvement. In the chronic stage, the small bowel develops submucosal thickening and adhesions and fistulae may develop. The most common cause of radiation enteritis is pelvic radiotherapy for gynaecological malignancy or rectal cancer.

Chapman & Nakielny, *Aids to Radiological Differential Diagnosis*, pp 140–141.

QUESTION 28

ANSWER: D

There is considerable overlap in the imaging appearances of these two conditions, but punctate calcification occurs in over half of patients with fibrolamellar carcinoma and is extremely unusual in FNH.

Reference: *Grainger & Allison's* 5e, pp 739–749.

QUESTION 29

ANSWER: D

High-frequency endosonography allows an accurate assessment of the four layers of the anal wall; superficial and deep mucosa, submucosa and muscularis propria.

Reference: *Grainger & Allison's* 5e, pp 681–682, 703.

QUESTION 30

ANSWER: B

Involvement of the GI tract is not uncommon in endometriosis and the sigmoid colon and pelvic small bowel loops are typical sites of involvement.

Reference: *Grainger & Allison's* 5e, p 701.

QUESTION 31

ANSWER: D

Oesophagectomy may be performed by a transhiatal approach or by thoracotomy, depending on the location of the tumour and condition of the patient (a posterior rib resection is a useful radiographic clue). In this patient, it is likely that a 'neo-oesophagus' has been formed by anastomosing the oesophageal remnant with the stomach in the upper chest. The neo-oesophagus will appear as a paramediastinal soft tissue density mass on plain radiographs and may contain an air:fluid level. The presence of a hydropneumothorax at this stage suggests anastomotic leakage and is a significant abnormal finding.

Reference: Upponi S, Ganeshan A, Slater A, et al. Imaging following surgery for oesophageal cancer. *Clin Radiol* 2007;62:724–731.

QUESTION 32

ANSWER: B

The development of gas in the gallbladder of an unwell diabetic patient is suggestive of emphysematous cholecystitis.

Reference: *Grainger & Allison's* 5e, pp 769–772.

QUESTION 33

ANSWER: D

Ménétrier's disease characteristically produces thickened hyperplastic mucosa (sparing the gastric antrum) but the stomach remains pliable.

Reference: *Grainger & Allison's* 5e, p 637.

QUESTION 34

ANSWER: D

In peritoneal TB, the presence of dense ascites, peritoneal nodularity and lymph nodes with low attenuation centres are characteristic findings.

Reference: *Grainger & Allison's* 5e, pp 712–714.

QUESTION 35

ANSWER: C

A history of inflammatory bowel disease is associated with significantly increased risk of cholangiocarcinoma.

Reference: *Grainger & Allison's* 5e, pp 781–782.

QUESTION 36

ANSWER: C

Anastomotic leakage is one of the most serious complications following gastric surgery and may occur in the acute or chronic phase. In a contrast study, water-soluble contrast should be used initially, but if no leak is detected then barium can be used as it is more sensitive for the detection of subtle postoperative leaks (outweighing the risk of barium spilling into the peritoneal cavity). The most common site for leakage is at surgical anastomoses and suture lines; therefore control images are invaluable to note the location of these sites and look for extraluminal gas.

Reference: Woodfield CA, Levine MS. The postoperative stomach. *Eur J Radiol* 2005;53:341–352.

QUESTION 37

ANSWER: C

In Mirizzi syndrome, a gallstone in the cystic duct produces mass effect on the common duct and can lead to fistula formation.

Reference: *Grainger & Allison's* 5e, pp 777–779.

QUESTION 38

ANSWER: D

Ultrasound findings of acute cholecystitis also include gallbladder distension and the sonographic Murphy's sign (the patient is unable to breathe in deeply when the probe is pressed firmly over the gallbladder). The normal gallbladder wall can measure up to 3 mm in thickness and wall thickening may be due to nonbiliary causes (hypoalbuminaemia, heart failure, etc).

Reference: Chapman & Nakielny, *Aids to Radiological Differential Diagnosis*, p 171.

QUESTION 39

ANSWER: A

When contrast is injected into the hepatic veins, a 'spider's web' appearance of collateral vessels is diagnostic of Budd Chiari syndrome.

Reference: *Grainger & Allison's* 5e, pp 751–755.

QUESTION 40

ANSWER: A

Amiodarone contains iodine; therefore deposition in the liver leads to increased density on CT.

References: *Grainger & Allison's* 5e, p 733.
Chapman & Nakielny, *Aids to Radiological Differential Diagnosis*, p 175.

QUESTION 41

ANSWER: E

If the tumour is in contact with more than half of the vessel circumference, it is very unlikely to be resectable.

Reference: *Grainger & Allison's* 5e, pp 801–803.

QUESTION 42

ANSWER: C

A gallstone causing a cholecystoduodenal fistula and aerobilia can also obstruct the distal small bowel.

Reference: *Grainger & Allison's* 5e, p 771.

QUESTION 43

ANSWER: B

Care should be taken not to overfill the intrahepatic ducts as the patient can rapidly become haemodynamically unstable. Biliary sepsis is a relative contraindication to PTC but a drainage procedure may be required in the setting of an obstructed and infected biliary system. A plastic or metallic stent may be inserted to treat a biliary stricture, but metallic stents should only be used in inoperable tumours as they cannot be subsequently removed. PTC and biliary stenting is usually performed using sedation and local anaesthesia and prophylactic antibiotics are routinely administered, whether a diagnostic or therapeutic procedure is being performed.

Reference: Chapman S, Nakielny R. *A Guide to Radiological Procedures*, 4th edition (Edinburgh: Saunders, 2003), pp 115–121.

QUESTION 44

ANSWER: C

Known as the 'squeeze sign'.

Reference: *Grainger & Allison's* 5e, p 700.

QUESTION 45

ANSWER: C

Hepatic adenoma, HCC and focal nodular hyperplasia will usually show marked enhancement in the arterial phase. Hypervascular liver metastases are typically hypointense on T1, hyperintense on T2. The characteristic behaviour of a liver haemangioma—not HCC—is described in option E.

Reference: Yu SCH, Yeung DTK, So NMC. Imaging features of hepatocellular carcinoma *Clin Radiol* 2004;59:145–156

QUESTION 46

ANSWER: D

Previous splenic injury leads to autotransplantation of splenic tissue onto serosal surfaces within the abdomen.

Reference: *Grainger & Allison's* 5e, pp 1761–1769.

QUESTION 47

ANSWER: E

This rare condition is secondary to chronic inflammation causing dilated excretory ducts ('flask shaped' projections of barium) in the oesophageal wall.

Reference: *Grainger & Allison's* 5e, p 624.

QUESTION 48

ANSWER: A

Necrotic pancreatic tissue will demonstrate reduced or absent enhancement on contrast-enhanced CT. It may not be possible to differentiate sterile from infected necrosis, but the presence of gas is a strong predictor of infection. Local vascular complications are well recognised to occur in severe acute pancreatitis but may occur without pancreatic necrosis.

Reference: Saokar A, Rabinowitz CB, Sahani DV. Cross-sectional imaging in acute pancreatitis. *Radiol Clin North Am* 2007;45(3):447–460.

QUESTION 49

ANSWER: E

The cystic pancreatic lesion is likely to be a serous cystadenoma and, in combination with simple pancreatic and renal cysts, is consistent with VHL.

Reference: *Grainger & Allison's* 5e, pp 792, 804.

QUESTION 50

ANSWER: E

Up to 10% of patients with primary sclerosing cholangitis will develop cholangiocarcinoma.

Reference: *Grainger & Allison's* 5e, pp 777–778.

QUESTION 51

ANSWER: E

CT colonography (CTC) is accepted as a generally safe technique with a reported perforation rate in symptomatic patients of 0.03% (compared with 0.13% with optical colonoscopy). Supine and prone imaging is widely advocated in CTC to maximise colonic distension and discriminate between faecal/fluid bowel residue and genuine pathology, while the use of an antispasmodic is advised to avoid colonic spasm. There is no strong evidence that intravenous contrast improves detection of colonic lesions, but it may be of benefit in symptomatic patients as it enables a more accurate assessment of extracolonic pathology.

Reference: Tolan DJM, Armstrong EM, Burling D, et al. Optimization of CT colonography technique: a practical guide. *Clin Radiol* 2007;62:819–827.

QUESTION 52

ANSWER: A

The history is typical of acute diverticulitis. These CT findings would be consistent with 'moderate' diverticulitis with a small pericolonic abscess.

Reference: *Grainger & Allison's* 5e, pp 690–692.

QUESTION 53

ANSWER: D

Repeated swallowing can interrupt normal peristalsis and produce a falsely abnormal appearance.

Reference: *Grainger & Allison's* 5e, pp 610–611.

QUESTION 54

ANSWER: A

The presence of cyst-like gas pockets in the left hemicolon of a patient with COPD is suggestive of pneumatosis cystoides intestinalis (pneumatosis coli).

Reference: *Grainger & Allison's* 5e, pp 599–601.

QUESTION 55

ANSWER: B

This clinical history is classic for a Krukenberg tumour—ovarian metastases from a GI tumour (most frequently a gastric adenocarcinoma).
Colorectal cancer is the second most common cause of this type of metastatic tumour presentation. Although melanoma may spread anywhere in the body, it is not a common cause of ovarian metastases. Metastatic ovarian cancer is made less likely by the minimally elevated CA-125 (would expect very high levels) and the presence of liver metastases.

Reference: Yada-Hashimoto M, Yamato T, Kamiura S, et al. Metastatic ovarian tumors: a review of 64 cases. *Gynecol Oncol* 2003;89(2):314–317.

QUESTION 56

ANSWER: C

Barium sulphate preparations consist of tiny particles (less than 1 μm) in a nonionic suspension.

References: *Grainger & Allison's* 5e, p 660.
Chapman & Nakielny, *A Guide to Radiological Procedures*, 4th edition (Edinburgh: Saunders, 2003), pp 62–64.

QUESTION 57

ANSWER: D

Up to 5% of liver transplants develop PTLD: extranodal disease is the most common pattern.

Reference: *Grainger & Allison's* 5e, p 1754.

QUESTION 58

ANSWER: C

The patient is highly likely to be severely neutropenic at this stage and the CT findings are typical of neutropenic colitis.

Reference: *Grainger & Allison's* 5e, p 698.

QUESTION 59

ANSWER: D

The clinical and imaging findings are highly suggestive of Zollinger-Ellision syndrome (hyperaciditiy due to an underlying gastrinoma).

Reference: *Grainger & Allison's* 5e, p 804.

QUESTION 60

ANSWER: C

The Parks' classification defines anal fistulae by the structures involved.
The intersphincteric fistula is the most common of anal fistulae (around 70%)
and does not pass through the external sphincter. A trans-sphincteric fistula will
cross both the internal and external sphincters to reach the skin surface while a
suprasphincteric fistula passes above the puborectalis muscle to involve the
ischiorectal fossa. The least common fistula is the extrasphincteric fistula as this
arises from the rectum and passes through the levator ani muscles to reach the
skin surface without involving the anal sphincter mechanism at all.

Reference: *Grainger & Allison's* 5e, pp 703–704.

QUESTION 61

ANSWER: B

The right paracolic gutter communicates freely with the right perihepatic
space (bounded by the falciform ligament). Postoperative gallbladder
collections will tend to lie in the gallbladder fossa and the hepatorenal recess
(also known as Morrison's pouch).

Reference: *Grainger & Allison's* 5e, pp 707–708.

QUESTION 62

ANSWER: A

Colonic pseudo-obstruction can produce the same radiographic findings as
large bowel obstruction: an instant contrast enema or CT should differentiate
mechanical obstruction from pseudo-obstruction.

Reference: *Grainger & Allison's* 5e, pp 595–596.

QUESTION 63

ANSWER: C

In adults, a minority of Meckel's diverticula contain gastric mucosa and can lead to GI bleeding. The diverticulum may also become inverted and act as a 'lead point' for an intussusception.

References: *Grainger & Allison's* 5e, p 674.
Chapman & Nakielny, *Aids to Radiological Differential Diagnosis*, p 160.

QUESTION 64

ANSWER: D

In acute viral hepatitis, there can be diffusely reduced reflectivity of the liver but the majority of patients have a normal ultrasound examination.

Reference: *Grainger & Allison's* 5e, p 733.

QUESTION 65

ANSWER: B

The normal gallbladder will appear after approximately 20 minutes. In acute cholecystitis, the gallbladder is typically not seen due to cystic duct obstruction.

References: *Grainger & Allison's* 5e, p 769.
Chapman & Nakielny, *A Guide to Radiological Procedures*, 4th edition (Edinburgh: Saunders, 2003), pp 127–131.

QUESTION 66

ANSWER: B

Ascites can occur with other colitides, but is often seen in pseudomembranous colitis. CT typically demonstrates mucosal enhancement and marked colonic wall thickening but only mild pericolonic stranding, in patients with pseudomembranous colitis. These findings have a high positive predictive value but a normal CT does not exclude pseudomembranous colitis. Rectal sparing occurs in around 10% of patients.

Reference: Ramachandran I, Sinha R, Rodgers P. Pseudomembranous colitis revisited: spectrum of imaging findings. *Clin Radiol* 2006;61:535–544.

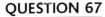

QUESTION 67

ANSWER: A

Gas, blood or flow voids can all produce filling defects in the biliary tree on MRCP.

Reference: *Grainger & Allison's* 5e, pp 766, 775–777.

QUESTION 68

ANSWER: C

The mid-oesophagus has the heart, pericardium and left main bronchus as its key anterior relations.

Reference: *Grainger & Allison's* 5e, p 609.

QUESTION 69

ANSWER: B

Torsion of an epiploic appendage leads to sudden onset of localised pain with characteristic CT findings of a pericolic inflammatory mass with central fat density.

Reference: *Grainger & Allison's* 5e, p 692.

QUESTION 70

ANSWER: A

Advanced gastric carcinoma is far more likely to directly invade local structures and obliterate the perigastric fat planes.

Reference: *Grainger & Allison's* 5e, pp 646–648.

QUESTION 71

ANSWER: A

The anterior pararenal space is the most anterior of the three retroperitoneal compartments.

Reference: *Grainger & Allison's* 5e, p 790.

QUESTION 72

ANSWER: B

In- and out-of-phase sequences utilise chemical shift artefact. Fat deposition in the liver will show a significant reduction in signal during the out-of-phase images.

Reference: *Grainger & Allison's* 5e, pp 95–98, 743.

QUESTION 73

ANSWER: C

Benign strictures in UC are typically smooth and symmetrical and are due to chronic smooth muscle hypertrophy. These occur in 10–20% of patients with UC and are most common in the left colon. Carcinomas arise from dysplastic changes within the diseased epithelium and not from adenomas as in the general population.

Reference: *Grainger & Allison's* 5e, pp 696, 699–700.

QUESTION 74

ANSWER: D

This angiographic finding is diagnostic of a Meckel's diverticulum as it indicates that a remnant of the omphalomesenteric (vitelline) duct is present.

Reference: *Grainger & Allison's* 5e, p 674.

QUESTION 75

ANSWER: D

The history of elevated CA 19–9 and obstructive jaundice is highly suggestive of a pancreatic ductal adenocarcinoma. The classic CT appearance of pancreatic ductal adenocarcinoma is a hypovascular mass with pancreatic and/or bile duct dilatation. Using a pancreatic mass protocol, these typical CT findings have a high positive predictive value and can help to differentiate ductal adenocarcinoma from other pancreatic masses (focal pancreatitis, neuroendocrine tumours, etc).

Reference: Amin Z, Theis B, Russell RCG, et al. Diagnosing pancreatic cancer: the role of percutaneous biopsy and CT. *Clin Radiol* 2006;61:996–1002.

QUESTION 76

ANSWER: B

The ultrasound findings are typical of pneumobilia. Other causes include an incompetent sphincter of Oddi (usually elderly patients) and a surgical procedure involving a Roux loop.

Reference: *Grainger & Allison's* 5e, pp 734–736.

QUESTION 77

ANSWER: C

A polyp will usually demonstrate uniform soft tissue density, similar to the surrounding bowel wall.

Reference: *Grainger & Allison's* 5e, pp 685–686.

QUESTION 78

ANSWER: A

Bowel wall thickening, lack of enhancement, adjacent fluid and pneumatosis intestinalis are all CT signs of ischaemia (strangulation) in small bowel obstruction. Fifty to 80% of small bowel obstruction is attributable to adhesions while 10% is due to hernias. In adhesions, there will usually be a history of previous abdominal surgery with CT demonstrating small bowel obstruction. The transition point may be identified, but the actual adhesive band is usually not visualised.

Reference: Qalbani A, Paushter D, Dachman AH. Multidetector row CT of small bowel obstruction. *Radiol Clin North Am* 2003;45(3):499–512.

QUESTION 79

ANSWER: A

The majority of symptomatic pancreatic cysts are pseudocysts; approximately one-half of pancreatic pseudocysts resolve spontaneously.

Reference: *Grainger & Allison's* 5e, pp 796–797, 808.

QUESTION 80

ANSWER: E

The combination of water-soluble contrast enema and CT is used to look for anastomotic leakage and abscess formation.

Reference: *Grainger & Allison's* 5e, p 702.

QUESTION 81

ANSWER: B

A gallbladder fossa mass with little/no visible normal gallbladder and hilar biliary obstruction is highly suggestive of gallbladder carcinoma.

References: *Grainger & Allison's* 5e, p 772.
Gore RM, Yaghmai V, Newmark GM, et al. Imaging benign and malignant disease of the gallbladder. *Radiol Clin North Am* 2002;40:1307–1323.

QUESTION 82

ANSWER: C

The body and tail of the pancreas lie posterior to the stomach and can be infiltrated by direct extension of a gastric tumour.

Reference: *Grainger & Allison's* 5e, pp 646–647.

QUESTION 83

ANSWER: E

An increased number of thickened valvulae conniventes are seen in the distal ileum with nodular filling defects due to lymphoid hyperplasia.

Reference: *Grainger & Allison's* 5e, p 671.

QUESTION 84

ANSWER: C

Calcification occurs in 2–3% of liver metastases. Mucinous adenocarcinoma of the GI tract is the most frequent underlying primary tumour.

Reference: *Grainger & Allison's* 5e, pp 750–751.

QUESTION 85

ANSWER: C

Stricture formation (with barium sacculation on double contrast enema) can occur in the splenic flexure due to fibrosis of the ischaemic bowel.

Reference: *Grainger & Allison's* 5e, pp 697–698.

QUESTION 86

ANSWER: B

A single 'giant' ulcer in an immunocompromised host is highly suggestive of a viral oesophagitis (eg CMV or herpes simplex).

Reference: *Grainger & Allison's* 5e, pp 623–624.

QUESTION 87

ANSWER: C

Extended echo times will emphasise the high T2 signal intensity of liver haemangiomas, in comparison with surrounding structures.

Reference: *Grainger & Allison's* 5e, pp 738–742.

QUESTION 88

ANSWER: D

The oesophagus is the most commonly involved part of the GI system in scleroderma. Oesophageal strictures can develop due to the severe reflux.

References: *Grainger & Allison's* 5e, p 623.
Chapman & Nakielny, *Aids to Radiological Differential Diagnosis*, pp 131–132.

QUESTION 89

ANSWER: B

Microbubble contrast agents act as positive contrast on ultrasound, and enhancement is seen as increasing echogenicity following contrast injection.

Reference: *Grainger & Allison's* 5e, pp 75-76, 745–748.

QUESTION 90

ANSWER: C

Intraductal calcification may be focal or diffuse and is not seen in all patients with chronic pancreatitis. When it is present, however, it is a highly reliable sign of chronic pancreatitis.

References: *Grainger & Allison's* 5e, pp 799–800.
Remer EM, Baker ME. Imaging of chronic pancreatitis. *Radiol Clin North Am* 2002;45:1229–1242.

QUESTION 91

ANSWER: E

Riedel's lobe is described as a 'tongue-like' projection of the anterior tip of the right lobe of liver. It is a variant of normal and is more common in women.

Reference: *Grainger & Allison's* 5e, p 726.

QUESTION 92

ANSWER: A

The majority of symptomatic cystic pancreatic lesions are pseudocysts and many will resolve spontaneously. Serous cystadenomas can occur anywhere in the pancreas and contain multiple small cysts measuring up to 20 mm each while up to one-third contain calcification. Ninety per cent of mucinous (macrocystic) cystadenomas occur in the pancreatic body and tail and the cysts typically measure greater than 20 mm. Long-term follow-up of cystic pancreatic lesions indicates that an asymptomatic simple cyst measuring less than 20 mm is unlikely to become clinically significant.

Reference: Planner AC, Anderson EM, Slater A, et al. An evidence-based review for the management of cystic pancreatic lesions. *Clin Radiol* 2007;62:930–937.

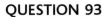

QUESTION 93

ANSWER: C

Iohexol is a widely used low osmolar contrast medium and does not confer increased risk of biliary tract malignancy. Previous exposure to Thorotrast (thorium dioxide) is a recognised risk factor, however.

References: *Grainger & Allison's* 5e, pp 781–782.
Baron RL, Tublin ME, Peterson MS. Imaging the spectrum of biliary tract disease. *Radiol Clin North Am* 2002;40:1325–1354.

QUESTION 94

ANSWER: B

The word desmoplastic comes from the Greek 'desmos' and 'plasty', meaning 'to form a band'. It describes the growth of fibrous bands infiltrating into adjacent tissue and is a recognised feature of GI carcinoid tumours.

Reference: *Grainger & Allison's* 5e, pp 667–669, 721–722.

QUESTION 95

ANSWER: A

Aphthous ulceration is the earliest sign of Crohn's disease on a double contrast barium enema. The other options are all true of ulcerative colitis—from the earliest signs of fine mucosal granularity to the 'lead pipe' appearance of the colon in chronic UC. Submucosal ulceration can extend laterally in UC giving the 'collar button' appearance.

Reference: Ambrosini R, Barchiesi A, De Mizio D, et al. Inflammatory disease of the colon: how to image. *Eur J Radiol* 2007;61:442–448.

QUESTION 96

ANSWER: C

The 'pseudotumour', 'pseudokidney' and 'target' signs all describe the characteristic sonographic appearance of intussusception.

Reference: *Grainger & Allison's* 5e, pp 595, 1499–1501.

QUESTION 97

ANSWER: D

An instant enema can exclude mechanical obstruction in patients with colonic pseudo-obstruction.

Reference: *Grainger & Allison's* 5e, pp 598–599.

QUESTION 98

ANSWER: A

Acalculous cholecystitis should always be considered in the seriously ill patient who develops unexplained sepsis.

Reference: *Grainger & Allison's* 5e, pp 770–771.

QUESTION 99

ANSWER: D

Melanoma metastases have a different appearance to most liver metastases as the paramagnetic effect of melanin leads to high T1 and low T2 signal.

References: *Grainger & Allison's* 5e, pp 746–748, 751.
Chapman & Nakielny, *Aids to Radiological Differential Diagnosis*, p 177.

QUESTION 100

ANSWER: D

Red cell scintigraphy is the most sensitive method of detecting active GI bleeding (catheter angiography can only detect bleeding of 0.5 ml/min).

Reference: *Grainger & Allison's* 5e, pp 578–580.

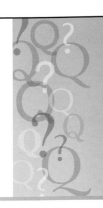

MODULE 4

Genitourinary, Adrenal, Obstetric & Gynaecology and Breast

QUESTIONS

QUESTION 1

A 48-year-old man presents with a painless swelling in the right scrotum. He has a past medical history of bilateral undescended testes and subsequent orchidopexy. On examination, there is a firm right testicular lump but no inguinal lymphadenopathy. On ultrasound, a well-defined, homogeneous hyporeflective mass was found within the right testicle. The right epididymis and contralateral testicle appeared normal. What is the most likely diagnosis?

  A Leukaemic testicular infiltrate
  B Testicular epidermoid cyst
  C Testicular metastasis
  D Testicular seminoma
  E Testicular teratoma

Answer on page 257

QUESTION 2

A 65-year-old man with transitional cell carcinoma of the bladder undergoes a pelvic MRI. On T1w sequences, there is a 2-cm papillary bladder wall growth that returns signal intensity higher than that of the surrounding urine and extends into the bladder wall. On T2w sequences, an uninterrupted low signal intensity line clearly separates the tumour from the surrounding perivesical fat. No perivesical stranding is seen. Which one of the following options best describes the staging of the tumour?

A T2a

B T2b

C T3a

D T3b

E T4a

Answer on page 257

QUESTION 3

A 65-year-old man is referred to the urology outpatient clinic with a painless right testicular lump. On ultrasound, there is a 3-cm heterogeneous mass within the right testicle that has concentric rings of alternating hypo- and hyperechogenicity, giving the mass a 'whorled' appearance. A subsequent MRI shows this mass to have alternating low and high signal intensity layers on T2w sequences. What is the most likely diagnosis?

A Melanoma metastases

B Orchitis

C Testicular abscess

D Testicular epidermoid cyst

E Testicular microlithiasis

Answer on page 258

QUESTION 4

A 13-year-old boy presents to the Emergency Department with sudden onset of left scrotal pain, fever and vomiting. The referring clinician suspects left testicular torsion and requests an urgent ultrasound prior to surgical exploration. Which of the following radiological findings would suggest that the left testis is still viable?

A A diffusely enlarged hypoechoic left testis

B A normal echogenicity testis on grey-scale imaging

C A small shrunken left testis with a surrounding hydrocoele and scrotal wall thickening

D Absent blood flow within the left testis on colour flow Doppler but good flow within the tunica vaginalis

E An enlarged heterogeneous left testis

Answer on page 258

QUESTION 5

A 25-year-old man presents with a tender right scrotum. Which one of the following statements best describes the expected ultrasound findings in acute, uncomplicated epididymo-orchitis?

A A small atrophic right testis

B A well-defined testicular mass of mixed echogenicity that has a whorled appearance and reduced flow on colour Doppler

C Multiple small (approx. 1 mm) echogenic foci scattered throughout the right testis

D Patchy areas of increased echogenicity within the testis with reduced flow on colour Doppler

E Well-defined, patchy areas of decreased echogenicity within the right testis

Answer on page 258

QUESTION 6

A 35-year-old man is discovered to have a right testicular mass on ultrasound. Which additional ultrasound finding would suggest a diagnosis of teratoma rather than seminoma?

A A testicular mass that contains areas of calcification

B A testicular mass that demonstrates increased colour Doppler flow

C A testicular mass that is homogeneously anechoic with posterior acoustic enhancement

D A testicular mass that is hypoechoic compared with the surrounding testicular parenchyma

E A testicular mass that has well-defined margins

Answer on page 258

QUESTION 7

A 32-year-old man received a cadaveric renal transplant 3 days ago. He now presents with increasing right iliac fossa pain and deteriorating renal function. On ultrasound, there is mild dilatation of the pelvicalyceal system with prominent renal pyramids. On Doppler ultrasound, colour Doppler flow is present within the renal artery and the interlobar arteries. The interlobar arterial waveform has tall systolic peaks with diastolic flow below the baseline. What is the most likely diagnosis?

A Acute tubular necrosis

B Acute rejection

C Arteriovenous fistula

D Renal artery stenosis at the site of anastomosis

E Renal vein thrombosis

Answer on page 259

QUESTION 8

A full-term neonate has a palpable left-sided abdominal mass. On ultrasound, the right kidney appears normal whilst the left kidney is grossly enlarged, containing multiple anechoic cysts of varying sizes which do not communicate with each other. A subsequent MAG3 scintigram confirms normal function within the right kidney and no evidence of isotope uptake on the left. What is the most likely underlying diagnosis?

 A Autosomal dominant polycystic kidney disease (ADPKD)
 B Autosomal recessive polycystic kidney disease (ARPKD)
 C Hydronephrosis
 D Infantile form of medullary sponge kidney (IMSK)
 E Multicystic dysplastic kidney disease (MCKD)

Answer on page 259

QUESTION 9

A 40-year-old male diabetic patient has an intravenous urogram (IVU) for left-sided renal colic. On the IVU, the left kidney shows papillary and calyceal abnormalities that give an 'egg in a cup' appearance at some calyces and 'tracks and horns' at other calyces. The affected left kidney has preserved renal cortical thickness despite the calyceal/papillary abnormalities. The contralateral kidney appears normal. What is the most likely diagnosis?

 A Acute pyelonephritis
 B Amyloidosis
 C Reflux nephropathy
 D Renal papillary necrosis
 E Xanthogranulomatous pyelonephritis

Answer on page 259

QUESTION 10

A 40-year-old female diabetic patient has right loin pain, vomiting and a fever. An ultrasound examination is requested to exclude urinary obstruction. This demonstrates no evidence of upper tract dilatation, but features of acute pyelonephritis are present. What are the most likely sonographic findings within the right kidney?

A Focal areas of reduced reflectivity in the renal parenchyma
B Focal atrophy of segments of the right kidney
C Increased echogenicity of the renal calyces
D Enlarged right kidney and diffusely hyperechoic parenchyma
E Shrunken right kidney and diffusely hyperechoic parenchyma

Answer on page 259

QUESTION 11

A 43-year-old female diabetic patient with right-sided renal colic has a CT urogram (CTU). This demonstrates a calculus within the right renal pelvis and the right renal cortex is almost entirely replaced by a heterogeneous ill-defined mass that extends to involve Gerota's fascia. This right renal mass contains rounded areas of low attenuation (-15 to -20 HU) which don't enhance postcontrast. On a subsequent MRI, the right renal mass appears heterogeneous with rounded areas of high signal on T1w and low signal on STIR images. What is the most likely diagnosis?

A Emphysematous pyelonephritis
B Renal angiomyolipoma
C Renal cell carcinoma
D Staghorn calculus with coexistent malakoplakia
E Xanthogranulomatous pyelonephritis.

Answer on page 260

QUESTION 12

A 58-year-old woman suffers a left ureteric injury during a total abdominal hysterectomy. Postoperatively, she develops left loin pain and a fever, and ultrasound demonstrates a moderate left hydronephrosis. The clinical team are concerned that she has an infected, obstructed left kidney and request a nephrostomy. Which one of the following statements is correct regarding percutaneous nephrostomy?

A A 4 French nephrostomy catheter is adequate to drain an infected collecting system likely to contain pus.

B If the renal pelvis is punctured with the wire during a successful procedure, the patient will always require surgical repair.

C It is best to dilate the tract 1 French size bigger than the size of the intended nephrostomy catheter (eg 8F for a 7F catheter).

D It is best to directly puncture the renal pelvis.

E It is usually best to aim to puncture an upper pole calyx.

Answer on page 260

QUESTION 13

A 55-year-old HIV-positive man presents with macroscopic haematuria and right-sided renal colic. An IVU does not demonstrate any renal tract calcification, but there is a dense right nephrogram with no excretion of contrast on a delayed film. The urologist performs a retrograde ureteroscopy and retrieves a 9-mm right ureteric calculus. What is the likely composition of the calculus?

A Calcium oxalate

B Cysteine

C Indinavir phosphate

D Struvite

E Uric acid

Answer on page 260

QUESTION 14

A 58-year-old man recently migrated to the UK from Kenya. He has been experiencing haematuria, weight loss and dysuria for several months. A series of imaging investigations are requested by the urologists and reveal evidence of renal tract TB. Which one of the following statements best describes the likely radiological findings in renal tract tuberculosis?

A A chest radiograph is normal in 75–80% of cases.

B Bladder calcification is more commonly seen than renal or ureteric calcification.

C Free vesicoureteric reflux into a widely dilated upper renal tract is frequently seen.

D Tramline calcification is seen within the seminal vesicles.

E Findings usually present as bilateral renal tract disease.

Answer on page 260

QUESTION 15

A 29-year-old man has an IVU performed following an episode of haematuria. This demonstrates complete right-sided ureteric duplication. Which one of the following statements is true?

A If present, an ectopic ureterocoele is usually related to the lower moiety ureter.

B The lower moiety ureter usually obstructs at the vesicoureteric junction.

C The upper moiety calyces are prone to vesicoureteric reflux.

D The upper moiety ureter is prone to ureteric obstruction.

E The upper moiety ureter usually inserts into the bladder superior to the lower moiety ureter.

Answer on page 261

QUESTION 16

A patient with normal renal function and suspected right renal artery stenosis undergoes a dynamic angiotensin converting enzyme inhibitor (ACEI) MAG3 renogram. Which one of the following statements best describes the findings of the ACEI renogram in right renal artery stenosis?

A After administration of the ACEI, there is increased blood flow to the right kidney.

B On a time activity graph, the mean transit time of the right kidney is reduced following ACEI.

C On a time activity graph, the time to peak of the right kidney is increased following ACEI.

D The ACEI renogram will be normal because the renal function is preserved.

E The ACEI renogram will show an increase in total and relative renal function of the right kidney when compared with the left kidney.

Answer on page 261

QUESTION 17

A 27-year-old man with membranous glomerulonephritis presents with a 1-day history of right-sided flank pain and haematuria. An abdominal radiograph did not reveal any renal calcification but his renal function has significantly deteriorated over the past 24 hours. On ultrasound there is a large, oedematous right kidney with loss of the corticomedullary differentiation. On a subsequent IVU, there is a faint nephrogram with absent pelvicalyceal filling after 15 minutes. What is the most likely diagnosis?

A Acute hydronephrosis

B Acute pyelonephritis

C Acute renal infarction

D Acute renal vein thrombosis

E Chronic pyelonephritis

Answer on page 261

QUESTION 18

A 37-year-old man presents with right flank pain, fever and tenderness. On a contrast-enhanced CT abdomen, there is a ring-enhancing mass just anterior to Gerota's fascia but posterior to the parietal peritoneum on the right. In which fascial compartment does the abnormality lie?

A Anterior pararenal space

B Anterior perinephric space

C Anterior subcapsular space

D Posterior pararenal space

E Posterior perinephric space

Answer on page 261

QUESTION 19

A 57-year-old diabetic man with a 6-week history of pyrexia of unknown origin has a contrast-enhanced CT abdomen. There is an upper pole renal mass that has a thick irregular enhancing wall with a central area of fluid attenuation with other areas of very low attenuation (-1000 HU). Which one of the following is the likely diagnosis?

A Metastatic disease

B Renal abscess

C Renal cyst with haemorrhage

D Renal infarction

E Renal lymphoma

Answer on page 261

QUESTION 20

A 74-year-old woman undergoes a follow-up CT for gastric carcinoma. She has previously received palliative chemotherapy, but has recently deteriorated with marked loss of weight. The CT demonstrates progressive disease with new lung and liver metastases and there are new abnormalities in both kidneys. Which one of the following statements best describes the CT findings of haematogenous metastases to the kidneys?

A Curvilinear (arc)-like calcification is a characteristic feature.

B Metastases to the kidney are usually < 3 cm in size and limited to the cortex.

C Multiple lesions involving the medulla are a feature of haematogenous metastases.

D If renal vein invasion is not present, renal metastases are highly unlikely.

E Renal metastases are usually hypovascular on contrast-enhanced CT.

Answer on page 262

QUESTION 21

A 41-year-old woman is diagnosed with significant right renal artery stenosis and referred for angioplasty. Regarding this procedure, which one of the following statements is correct?

A Angioplasty of ostial lesions has a poorer prognosis than angioplasty of more distal lesions.

B Intra-arterial GTN to treat vasospasm is contraindicated during the procedure.

C Stenoses due to fibromuscular dysplasia don't respond well to angioplasty alone.

D Stenoses due to fibromuscular dysplasia tend to involve the renal artery ostia.

E The majority of renal artery stenoses are due to fibromuscular dysplasia.

Answer on page 262

QUESTION 22

A 63-year-old nulliparous, obese female patient presents with postmenopausal bleeding. On a transvaginal ultrasound examination the endometrium is 8 mm thick. The radiology SpR suspects endometrial carcinoma and suggests an MRI for further evaluation. What MRI findings would support a diagnosis of endometrial carcinoma?

A On post-gadolinium T1w images, the thickened endometrium enhances less than the adjacent myometrium.

B On T1w sequences, the thickened abnormal endometrium appears hypointense to the adjacent myometrium.

C Post-gadolinium fat-suppressed T1w sequences show enhancement of the thickened endometrium.

D T1w sequences show the junctional zone as a low signal band sandwiched between the high signal endometrium and the intermediate signal peripheral myometrium.

E T2w sequences show the junctional zone as a high signal band.

Answer on page 262

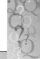

QUESTION 23

An 81-year-old woman presents to the Emergency Department with sepsis
and left iliac fossa pain. She has grossly elevated inflammatory markers
and serum creatinine = 212μmol/L. A contrast-enhanced CT is requested
for suspected acute diverticulitis, but the on-call radiology SpR is concerned
about the possibility of contrast-mediated nephrotoxicity (CMN). Which one
of the following statements is true regarding CMN?

A Atrial fibrillation is an independent risk factor for developing CMN.

B CMN is defined as renal impairment (an increase in serum creatinine by
more than 50% or by 44 μmol/L above baseline) within 24 hours of contrast injection.

C Low osmolar contrast media is more nephrotoxic than high osmolar
contrast media, in patients with pre-existing renal impairment.

D Pre-hydration with 1 mL/kg body weight/h of 0.9% NaCl for 4 hours
prior to the contrast injection may increase the incidence of CMN.

E Prophylactic haemodialysis in patients with renal impairment does not
reduce the risk of CMN.

Answer on page 262

QUESTION 24

A 64-year-old man presents with right renal colic and a kidney ureter bladder plain radiograph (CT KUB) is performed. This demonstrates an incidental 2-cm solid right adrenal mass. On the unenhanced CT, the mass is homogeneous and has an average density of 7 HU. What is the most likely diagnosis?

A Adrenal adenoma
B Adrenal hyperplasia
C Adrenal metastasis
D Focal adrenal haemorrhage
E Primary adrenal malignancy

Answer on page 263

QUESTION 25

A 62-year-old man has an MRI pelvis for biopsy-proven prostate cancer. Following thorough review of the examination, the reporting radiologist concludes that the patient's disease stage is T3N0M0. Which one of the following findings was likely to have been present on MRI?

A The prostatic capsule is breached with seminal vesicle invasion.
B Regional nodes > 10 mm in size.
C Tumour extends into both lobes of the prostate.
D Tumour involves only one lobe.
E Tumour invades the bladder neck.

Answer on page 263

QUESTION 26

A 36-year-old woman undergoes a pelvic MRI following the discovery of a left ovarian mass on ultrasound. The reporting radiologist identifies a 3-cm mass in the left ovary and believes this to be an ovarian fibroma. Which one of the following statements best describes the likely MRI findings?

A A left ovarian mass of high signal on T1w and low signal on T2w images

B A left ovarian mass of high signal on T1w, showing loss of signal on STIR images

C A left ovarian mass of high signal on T2w but low signal on T1w images

D A left ovarian mass yielding low signal on both T1w and T2w images

E Compared with in-phase images, the 3-cm ovarian mass shows signal loss in out-of-phase T1w sequences

Answer on page 263

QUESTION 27

Dynamic contrast-enhanced CT may be used to characterise adrenal lesions. Which one of the following statements best describes the imaging characteristics of a primary adrenal carcinoma on portal venous phase (70 s) and subsequent delayed phase (15 min) contrast-enhanced CT images?

A Early washout on delayed images

B No measurable enhancement in either phase

C Poor early enhancement, with an increase in enhancement on delayed images

D Washout by greater than 80%, compared with the early postcontrast images

E Washout of less than 40% on delayed images, compared with the portal venous phase images

Answer on page 264

QUESTION 28

You are the radiology SpR consenting a 70-year-old man for a transrectal ultrasound (TRUS) prostate biopsy. Which one of the following is not a recognised complication of this procedure?

A Haematuria

B Haematospermia

C Perirectal bleeding

D Pneumoperitoneum

E Pain/discomfort post-procedure

Answer on page 264

QUESTION 29

A 35-year-old patient received a cadaveric renal transplant 5 days ago and now presents with worsening renal function and decreasing urine output. Which one of the following findings on a Tc-99m DTPA radionuclide scan would favour a diagnosis of acute tubular necrosis (ATN) over acute rejection?

A Delayed renal excretion

B Elevated resistive index greater than 0.7

C Increased renal perfusion after administration of an ACEI (eg Captopril)

D Poor/impaired graft perfusion

E Preserved renal transplant perfusion

Answer on page 264

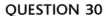

QUESTION 30

Which one of the following radiological findings is a recognised feature of Von Hippel Lindau (VHL) disease?

A Bilateral adrenal masses that yield a high signal on T2w sequences
B Cerebral aneurysms on CT angiography
C Evidence of calcified subependymal nodules on CT head
D Polymicrogyria and corpus callosum agenesis on MRI brain
E Unenhanced CT head demonstrating a midline, hyperdense vermian mass abutting the roof of the 4th ventricle

Answer on page 265

QUESTION 31

A 34-year-old man is knocked off his bicycle by a car and presents to the Emergency Department with bruising over the right flank and gross haematuria. The A&E SpR suspects renal injury and requests a CT abdomen. Which one of the following findings is most likely to be seen in uncomplicated renal contusion (Grade 1 renal injury)?

A Ill-defined areas of low attenuation with irregular margins
B Subcapsular high attenuation collection
C Wedge-shaped areas of high attenuation, typically involving the renal poles
D Well-defined areas of low attenuation within the renal parenchyma
E Urinoma formation

Answer on page 265

QUESTION 32

A 24-year-old motorcyclist involved in a traffic accident presents to the Emergency Department with a broken leg and bruising over his left flank. He is found to have microscopic haematuria and fractures of the left 8th and 9th ribs. The patient is haemodynamically stable and clinicians suspect a left renal injury. Which one of the following imaging investigations is the most appropriate?

A Abdominal ultrasound
B Contrast-enhanced CT abdomen and pelvis
C Emergency catheter renal angiography
D Gadolinium-enhanced renal MRI
E IVU

Answer on page 265

QUESTION 33

A 22-year-old woman is kicked in the abdomen during an attempted robbery. She presents with haematuria and a triple-phase CT abdomen (arterial, portal venous and delayed phases) shows a left ureteric injury. What level is the ureteric injury most likely to be at?

A At the level of the ischial spines
B Lower third of the ureter
C Middle third of the ureter
D Pelviureteric junction
E Vesicoureteric junction

Answer on page 265

QUESTION 34

A 68-year-old man is involved in a traffic accident and sustains a pelvic fracture, head and limb injuries. Attempted urethral catheterisation in the Emergency Department is unsuccessful and a cystourethrogram is requested to exclude urethral injuries. Regarding urethral injuries, which one of the following statements is correct?

A Anterior urethral injury is more commonly due to iatrogenic or penetrating trauma than to blunt trauma.

B Cystography should precede a retrograde urethrogram in a patient with suspected urethral injury.

C In men, on digital rectal examination the prostate is lower than normal in patients with urethral trauma.

D Urethral injuries occur in 50% of major pelvic fractures.

E Urethral injury due to blunt trauma more commonly affects the penile urethra.

Answer on page 265

QUESTION 35

A 24-year-old motorcyclist is involved in a high-speed accident and is brought to the Emergency Department. He has abdominal guarding and is haemodynamically unstable. An ultrasound abdomen performed in the Emergency Department demonstrates free peritoneal fluid and a laparotomy is performed. In addition to liver and splenic lacerations, the surgeon finds a left retroperitoneal haematoma. Postoperatively, the on-call urologist requests a CT abdomen to assess the left renal injury. Which one of the following findings would indicate a Grade 4 renal laceration?

A Extravasation of contrast from the pelvicalyceal system on delayed phase (5 min) images

B Large (2-cm) subcapsular haematoma

C Perinephric haematoma that extends into the pararenal spaces

D Ill-defined low attenuation change in the lower pole renal cortex

E Segmental renal infarction

Answer on page 266

QUESTION 36

A 54-year-old man attends the Radiology Department for an ascending urethrogram. He has a past history of previous urethral stricture and urethroplasty at a different hospital and has now developed recurrent lower urinary tract symptoms. Which one of the following statements regarding urethral strictures is true?

A Inflammatory strictures most commonly occur within the penile urethra, the site of the periurethral glands.

B Most inflammatory strictures occur in the prostatic urethra.

C The urethral strictures due to transurethral retrograde prostatectomy (TURP) are typically long segment, irregular strictures.

D Traumatic strictures usually take longer to develop than inflammatory strictures.

E Ultrasound is more accurate than conventional urethrography in the assessment of urethral strictures.

Answer on page 266

QUESTION 37

Which one of the following statements best describes the radiological appearances of a parapelvic renal cyst?

A It does not opacify during IVU.

B If hydronephrosis is present, a parapelvic cyst can be excluded.

C It shows delayed (10 min) filling on IVU.

D It may have similar appearances to calyceal diverticula on IVU.

E The majority arise from the lower renal pole.

Answer on page 266

QUESTION 38

A 64-year-old man has an abdominal MRI to further characterise a well-defined 2.5-cm solid renal mass at the left upper pole. The lesion was hyperechoic on ultrasound. Which one of the following MRI findings would favour a diagnosis of angiomyolipoma?

A High signal on T1w and low signal on T2w sequences

B High signal on T1w and STIR sequences

C High signal on T1w and T2w sequences

D High signal on T2w and low signal on proton density sequences

E Low signal on both T2w and proton density sequences

Answer on page 266

QUESTION 39

A 42-year-old man is referred for investigation of painless microscopic haematuria. An IVU is performed and demonstrates bilateral small areas of calcification within the kidneys on the control image. On the 5-min postcontrast IVU film, the calcification appears to lie within the collecting system. On ultrasound, there are numerous small hyperechoic rounded areas within the medullary pyramids, many of which cast an acoustic shadow. What is the most likely diagnosis?

A Adult polycystic kidney disease

B Hyperparathyroidism

C Medullary sponge kidney

D Primary hyperoxaluria

E Sarcoidosis

Answer on page 267

QUESTION 40

A 36-year-old woman presents with primary infertility. A transabdominal ultrasound shows a normal anteverted uterus and bilateral adnexal masses. A subsequent MRI shows bilateral high signal ovarian masses on both T1w and T2w sequences. On fat-suppressed T1w images, the lesions remain high signal. What is the most likely diagnosis?

A Bilateral dermoid cysts
B Bilateral endometriomas
C Bilateral ovarian fibromas
D Bilateral theca lutein cysts
E Polycystic ovaries

Answer on page 267

QUESTION 41

A 32-year-old man involved in a high-speed traffic accident is found to have blood at the urethral meatus and a high riding prostate during the secondary clinical survey. The examining doctor suspects a urethral injury. Which part of the urethra is most likely to be involved?

A Bulbar urethra
B Membranous urethra
C Penile urethra
D Penoscrotal urethra
E Prostatic urethra

Answer on page 267

QUESTION 42

You are the radiologist reviewing the mammograms of a 56-year-old woman. When compared with her previous mammograms, areas of calcification previously seen within the left upper outer quadrant have now disappeared. Which of the following is not a possible explanation?

A Breast surgery

B Chemotherapy

C Postmenopausal changes

D Radiotherapy

E Spontaneous resolution

Answer on page 267

QUESTION 43

Which one of the following statements best describes the CT appearances of a renal oncocytoma (tubular adenoma)?

A It appears as a small, ill-defined renal mass in the majority of cases.

B It is bilateral in 60-80% of cases.

C It characteristically consists of multiple renal lesions.

D CT shows punctuate calcification in the majority of patients.

E Low attenuation (−100 to −50 HU) areas within a large lesion are consistent with an oncocytoma.

Answer on page 267

QUESTION 44

A 45-year-old woman presents with a 1-year history of menorrhagia.
On physical examination, her GP palpates a mass arising from the pelvis and
suspects uterine fibroids. The GP refers her for imaging to confirm the
diagnosis of uterine fibroids. Which one of the following radiological findings
would support this diagnosis?

A On T2w images, a well-circumscribed myometrial mass that is of
lower signal than the surrounding myometrium

B On ultrasound, multiple theca lutein cysts and an enlarged uterus that
contains multiple cystic areas

C On T1w images, a well-circumscribed high signal intensity mass arising
from the myometrium

D On postcontrast T1w images, a well-circumscribed, uniformly
enhancing myometrial mass that is of higher signal than the surrounding
myometrium

E Widened junctional zone on T1w images of the uterus.

Answer on page 268

QUESTION 45

A transvaginal ultrasound is performed on a 36-year-old woman with
dysfunctional uterine bleeding. This demonstrates an enlarged globular uterus
with a heterogeneous appearance of the myometrium. The myometrium
contains diffuse echogenic nodules, subendometrial echogenic linear striations
and 2- to 6-mm subendometrial cysts. Colour Doppler demonstrates a
speckled pattern of increased vascularity within the heterogeneous area of
myometrium. What is the most likely diagnosis?

A Adenomyosis

B Endometrial polyposis

C Gestational trophoblastic disease (GTD)

D Stage 1A endometrial cancer

E Uterine fibroid

Answer on page 268

QUESTION 46

A 52-year-old postmenopausal woman presents for her first screening mammogram. Within the right upper outer quadrant, there is a 2-cm well-defined, oval mass that has dense 'popcorn' calcification within it and is surrounded by a thin radiolucent rim. On ultrasound, the mass is well defined and hyperechoic with areas of acoustic shadowing due to contained calcification. What is the most likely diagnosis?

A Fat necrosis

B Fibroadenoma

C Hamartoma

D Oil cyst

E Papilloma

Answer on page 268

QUESTION 47

A 54-year-old man has an abdominal ultrasound that shows a 3-cm hyperechoic lesion at the upper pole of the left kidney. An unenhanced CT abdomen is subsequently performed and demonstrates a left upper pole heterogeneous renal mass with central areas of low attenuation (5–10 HU). After intravenous contrast is administered, this mass enhances by more than 30 HU. What is the most likely diagnosis?

A Angiomyolipoma

B Oncocytoma

C Renal abscess

D Renal cell carcinoma

E Unilocular renal cyst

Answer on page 268

QUESTION 48

A 60-year-old nulliparous woman presents with postmenopausal bleeding. On transvaginal ultrasound, her endometrium is 8 mm thick and the endomyometrial junction appeared indistinct. The radiologist suspects invasive endometrial cancer and refers her for an MRI examination. What are the likely findings on MRI?

A On unenhanced T1w images the endometrial cancer appears of high signal intensity compared to the surrounding myometrium.

B On contrast-enhanced T1w images, endometrial cancer shows avid enhancement compared with surrounding myometrium.

C On T2w images the normally high signal junctional zone is disrupted.

D T1w fat-saturated sequences are best used to assess the junctional zone.

E The endometrial cancer demonstrates delayed/little enhancement compared to the normal surrounding myometrium on postcontrast T1w images.

Answer on page 268

QUESTION 49

A 56-year-old woman is found to have a screen-detected breast cancer on her second screening mammogram. Two breast radiologists both agree that there is no evidence of malignancy on the previous mammograms, even in retrospect. Which one of the following statement best describes this interval cancer?

A An interval cancer has a better prognosis, when compared with other screen detected cancers.

B This is known as a Type 1 interval cancer.

C This is known as a Type 2a interval cancer.

D This is known as a Type 2b interval cancer.

E This is known as a Type 3 interval cancer.

Answer on page 269

QUESTION 50

A 42-year-old man with known Wegener's granulomatosis develops haematuria. He has an abdominal ultrasound which reveals small, smooth kidneys with diffuse thinning of the renal parenchyma. The pelvicalyceal systems appear normal but there is an increased amount of renal sinus fat. What is the most likely diagnosis?

A Bilateral vesicoureteric reflux
B Chronic glomerulonephritis
C Medullary sponge kidney
D Pyelonephritis
E Renal tuberculosis

Answer on page 269

QUESTION 51

A 22-year-old pregnant woman (30 weeks' gestation) presents with right flank pain. She has an abdominal ultrasound which shows dilatation of the right pelvicalyceal system. Which one of the following additional findings would suggest a diagnosis of mechanical ureteric obstruction rather than pregnancy-related dilatation?

A An elevated resistive index (RI)
B Decreased corticomedullary differentiation
C Hyperechoic renal parenchyma
D Renal parenchymal thinning
E Ureteric and pelvicalyceal dilatation

Answer on page 269

QUESTION 52

On a T2w MRI pelvis of a normal patient, the wall of the urinary bladder has an apparent dark band along its lateral wall on one side, with a bright band on the opposing lateral wall. Which one of the following accounts for this radiological appearance?

A A large flip angle
B Beam hardening artefact
C Chemical shift artefact
D Movement artefact in the phase-encoding direction
E Movement artefact in the slice select gradient

Answer on page 269

QUESTION 53

A 29-year-old man presents with a 4-hour history of sudden onset right loin pain, radiating to the right groin. The clinicians request an emergency IVU for suspected acute urinary obstruction. Which one of the following IVU features would be most consistent with acute urinary obstruction?

A Absent right nephrogram and no evidence of contrast excretion on the right
B An increasingly dense right nephrogram that remains present after 6 hours
C An initially dense right nephrogram, which then resolves within 30 minutes
D The right kidney being 10% longer than the left kidney
E The right kidney being small with an irregular cortical surface

Answer on page 269

QUESTION 54

A 35-year-old woman presents with a painless lump in the outer upper quadrant of her left breast. She is referred for an ultrasound examination of the left breast. Which of the following ultrasound findings would suggest a malignant rather than a benign breast mass?

A A larger transverse than anterior-to-posterior diameter

B Ill-defined echogenic halo around the lesion

C Less than 1 cm in greatest diameter

D Posterior acoustic enhancement

E Uniform hyperechogenicity

Answer on page 270

QUESTION 55

Which one of the following statements best describes the course of the normal ureter within the pelvis?

A Anterior to the inferior pubic ramus, the ureter runs posteromedially to enter the urinary bladder.

B In females, the ureter lies within the broad ligament where it is intra-peritoneal for a short portion of its length and runs inferomedially to enter the urinary bladder.

C In males, the ureter runs anterior to the cremasteric artery and turns medially to enter the urinary bladder.

D In the region of the ischial spine, the ureter turns medially, anteriorly and inferiorly to enter the bladder.

E The ureter enters the pelvis by crossing the bifurcation of the common iliac artery and runs medially to enter the urinary bladder.

Answer on page 270

QUESTION 56

An immunosuppressed 24-year-old man presents with left renal colic. He is referred for an IVU. The control film shows a gas containing, round lamellated mass within the urinary bladder. Postcontrast, there are multiple filling defects within the urinary bladder. What is the most likely cause of these appearances?

A Blood clot
B Bladder calculi
C Cystitis
D Fungal ball
E Schistosomiasis

Answer on page 270

QUESTION 57

A 67-year-old man with a history of transitional cell carcinoma of the bladder now presents with several episodes of haematuria. A cystoscopy and biopsies performed 4 weeks ago were negative and he now attends for an MRI pelvis. On sagittal T2w images, there is an area of thickening in the bladder wall with low signal change in the surrounding perivesical fat. Which one of the following findings would suggest a diagnosis of postbiopsy change, rather than recurrent transitional cell carcinoma?

A On dynamic contrast-enhanced T1w images, the area of low signal shows early and avid contrast enhancement.
B On fat-suppressed proton density sequences, this area returns a high signal.
C On post-gadolinium T1w images, inflammatory change avidly enhances whilst transitional cell carcinoma does not.
D The area shows delayed enhancement on T1w post-gadolinium images.
E There is signal loss on gradient echo images, due to tissue inhomogeneity.

Answer on page 270

QUESTION 58

A 53-year-old woman is recalled to the screening breast outpatient clinic as her initial mammograms have revealed an area of suspected microcalcification. Compared with the standard mammographic projections, which one of the following statements best describes the technique needed to provide magnification views?

A A double-coated film is necessary to avoid parallax and crossover.

B A molybdenum target is used because it provides a low energy spectrum.

C A smaller focal spot of 0.1 mm is used.

D An air gap is avoided as it reduces signal to noise ratio.

E Tube current should be as high as possible to keep exposure times short.

Answer on page 271

QUESTION 59

Which of the following best describes the radiological findings of urinary tract malakoplakia?

A Intramural bladder wall gas

B Multiple filling defects in the pelvicalyceal systems and proximal ureters on IVU, with sparing of the urinary bladder

C Multiple small oval filling defects at the bladder base

D Plaque-like thickening of the pelvicalyceal urothelium

E Tram-track calcification within the bladder wall

Answer on page 271

QUESTION 60

A 70-year-old man with prostate cancer has an MRI examination to locally stage the disease. In which part of the prostate gland is a carcinoma most likely to arise?

A Central zone

B Peripheral zone

C Peri-urethral zone

D Transitional zone

E Within the verumontanum

Answer on page 271

QUESTION 61

A 53-year-old woman is invited to attend a mobile breast screening unit for routine screening mammograms. Which one of the following statements is correct regarding the standard mammographic projections (the mediolateral oblique (MLO) and craniocaudal (CC) views)?

A A well-positioned CC view usually contains all the breast tissue.

B A well-positioned MLO view rarely shows the nipple in profile because of the oblique compression.

C On a well-positioned MLO the nipple should be at the lower border of the pectoralis minor.

D The MLO view is taken with the radiograph beam directed from superomedial to inferolateral.

E The pectoralis major muscle is demonstrated at the posterior border of a CC view in approximately 70% of individuals.

Answer on page 271

QUESTION 62

A 24-year-old man presents to his GP with increased urinary frequency. Physical examination is normal and he is referred for ultrasound. Transabdominal ultrasound demonstrates a cystic structure posterior to the urinary bladder and a TRUS is performed for further evaluation. TRUS reveals a midline anechoic structure in the posterior portion of the prostate gland, superior to the verumontanum. It does not communicate with either the bladder or the seminal vesicles. Which of the following is the most likely diagnosis?

A Bladder diverticulum

B External iliac artery aneurysm

C Mullerian duct cyst

D Seminal vesicle cyst

E Urethral cyst

Answer on page 272

QUESTION 63

A 53-year-old man has an MRI of his pelvis as a staging investigation for bladder cancer. The request card also states that the prostate is mildly enlarged on digital rectal examination and the serum prostate specific antigen (PSA) level is borderline elevated. The reporting radiologist reviews the prostate in detail. Which one of the following statements best describes the MRI findings of a normal prostate gland?

A On T1w images, the central zone is of higher signal intensity than the peripheral zone.

B On T1w images, the central zone is of lower signal intensity than the peripheral zone.

C On T2w images, the peripheral zone is of lower signal intensity than the central and transitional zones

D The peripheral zone is of higher signal intensity than the central zone on T2w images.

E The seminal vesicles are hypointense on T2w images.

Answer on page 272

QUESTION 64

Regarding the radiological anatomy of the normal prostate gland, which of the following statements is correct?

A The anterior fibromuscular band separates the prostate from the rectum.

B The central zone atrophies with advancing age.

C The neurovascular bundles lie anterolateral to the prostate gland.

D The prostate gland is a flattened conical structure with its apex pointed superiorly.

E The zonal anatomy of the adult prostate gland is seen on transabdominal ultrasound.

Answer on page 272

QUESTION 65

A 34-year-old man has recently completed his third cycle of chemotherapy for testicular cancer. He now presents with fever, chills and dysuria. Unenhanced CT of the pelvis shows two well-defined areas of low attenuation within the prostatic parenchyma. Following intravenous contrast, the normal prostate gland enhances whilst the low attenuation areas remain unchanged. In addition, there is some stranding within the periprostatic fat. What is the most likely diagnosis?

A Corpora amylacea

B Prostatic abscess

C Prostatic calculi

D Prostatic cancer

E Prostatic cysts

Answer on page 272

QUESTION 66

A 62-year-old patient with transitional cell bladder carcinoma has an MRI scan to locally stage the disease. Which of the following MRI findings would indicate invasion of the seminal vesicles?

A Decreased signal of the seminal vesicles on T1w images

B Increased signal of the seminal vesicles on T1w images

C Increased signal of the seminal vesicles on T2w images

D Obliteration of the angle between the seminal vesicles and the posterior bladder wall

E Reduction in size of the seminal vesicles

Answer on page 273

QUESTION 67

A 64-year-old woman with bladder cancer is discussed in the urology multidisciplinary meeting. A recent CT suggested the possibility of tumour extension into the perivesical fat and the urologists request an MRI pelvis to assess whether the bladder wall is breached (as this would upstage the tumour). Which one of the following MRI sequences is best for assessing bladder wall integrity?

A Gradient echo sequences with a long flip angle

B Postcontrast STIR

C Proton density fat saturation

D T1w (precontrast)

E T2w

Answer on page 273

QUESTION 68

A final year medical student attends a breast screening outpatient clinic as part of her clinical attachment. She wishes to know more about the UK NHS Breast Screening programme and asks several questions of the radiology SpR in the breast clinic. Which one of the following statements is true?

A Double reading of all screening mammograms must be performed.

B Incident screens may be performed using only the MLO view.

C The acceptance rate of women invited to breast screening is over 90%.

D Up to 20% of women are recalled from screening for further assessment.

E Women over 70 years of age may stay in the Breast Screening Programme by choice.

Answer on page 273

QUESTION 69

A 22-year-old woman presents to her GP with irregular menstrual periods. She is overweight with a body mass index of 32 and has excess body hair. Her LH/FSH ratio is elevated and her GP refers her for a pelvic ultrasound. Which one of the following findings are most likely to be present on ultrasound?

A Enlarged, oedematous ovaries with multiple packed follicles and pelvic-free fluid

B Enlarged ovaries with multiple peripheral cysts

C Normal appearances of the ovaries

D Ovarian mass with mixed cystic and solid components

E Ovaries replaced by multiple large cysts

Answer on page 273

QUESTION 70

A 33-year-old man presents with left renal colic. An abdominal radiograph is normal but a subsequent CT urogram demonstrates an obstructing, opaque 10-mm distal left ureteric calculus. What is the renal calculus most likely to be composed of?

A Calcium oxalate
B Calcium phosphate
C Cysteine
D Pure matrix
E Uric acid

Answer on page 274

QUESTION 71

A 74-year-old man with increased urinary frequency and hesitancy is found to have an enlarged prostate on digital rectal examination. He is referred for a TRUS and biopsy. Which one of the following statements best describes the TRUS findings of benign prostatic hypertrophy (BPH)?

A Dense echogenic foci are seen at the margin of the peripheral and transitional zones.
B The central zone is enlarged.
C The peripheral zone is enlarged and appears homogeneously hypoechoic.
D The peripheral zone is enlarged and is of mixed echogenicity.
E The transitional zone is enlarged.

Answer on page 274

QUESTION 72

A 24-year-old man sustains blunt trauma to the lower abdomen during a traffic accident. After initial resuscitation, he is haemodynamically stable but there is clinical suspicion of urinary bladder rupture. Which one of the following radiological findings on a retrograde cystogram would support intraperitoneal rather than extraperitoneal bladder rupture?

A Contrast extravasation which spreads out in a streaky, irregular manner
B Elliptical extravasation adjacent to the bladder neck
C Gas within the bladder
D Pelvic fracture
E Tear at the bladder dome

Answer on page 274

QUESTION 73

A 64-year-old woman presents with bloating and vague pelvic pain and is referred for a pelvic ultrasound. On transabdominal ultrasound, she is found to have a large right adnexal mass. Which one of the following sonographic findings would indicate that this mass is more likely to be malignant than benign?

A Doppler waveform with a high resistive index (> 0.8)
B Homogeneously hypoechoic mass with posterior acoustic enhancement
C Multiple septations that are approximately 1 mm thick
D Papillary projections
E Size > 4 cm

Answer on page 274

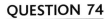

QUESTION 74

A 31-year-old woman has a hysterosalpingogram (HSG) as part of a series of investigations for primary infertility. The HSG shows a single vagina, single cervix but two separate uterine cavities leading to separate uterine horns. What is the most likely diagnosis?

A Arcuate uterus

B Bicornuate uterus

C Didelphus uterus

D Septate uterus

E Bicornis bicollis

Answer on page 274

QUESTION 75

A 67-year-old man attends the Emergency Department with acute abdminal pain. A CT abdomen is performed and demonstrates an uncomplicated acute appendicitis. The reporting radiologist notes an incidental finding of a bulky prostate gland. On axial CT images, which one of the following CT findings is an unequivocal feature of prostatic enlargement?

A The diaphragmatic urethra is dilated. (Dilatation)

B The prostate is identified 1 cm above the symphysis pubis.

C The prostate is identified 1 cm or less below the symphysis pubis.

D The prostate is identified 2–3 cm above the symphysis pubis.

E The prostate is identified less than 2 cm from the posterior aspect of the symphysis pubis.

Answer on page 275

QUESTION 76

A 65-year-old man is referred by his GP to the urologists for investigation of chronic macroscopic haematuria. The patient is a teacher and has recently returned to the UK after 15 years working in Malawi. He suffered an episode of dysuria and haematuria several years ago and a local doctor diagnosed schistosomiasis. You are asked to supervise and report a CT urogram for this patient. Which one of the following statements is true regarding the radiological features of schistosomiasis?

A Cortical nephrocalcinosis is characteristic.

B In late stage disease, a 1- to 3-mm band of calcification surrounding the bladder wall is seen.

C In the late stage, the bladder is dilated, thin walled and calcified, giving an egg-shell appearance.

D Narrowed 'pipe-stem' ureters are evident.

E 'Tram-line' calcification within the seminal vesicles is found in the majority of cases.

Answer on page 275

QUESTION 77

A 25-year-old man is seen in the Emergency Department following a fall from a height of 20 feet. Plain radiographs reveal a fractured pelvis and a cystogram is performed by the on-call radiology SpR. This demonstrates contrast extravasation from the urinary bladder in an irregular streaky fashion. Which one of the following is the most likely diagnosis?

A Bladder wall contusion

B Extraperitoneal bladder rupture

C Intraperitoneal bladder rupture

D Mixed intra- and extraperitoneal bladder rupture

E Subserosal bladder rupture

Answer on page 275

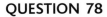

QUESTION 78

A 70-year-old man with urinary frequency and urge incontinence is referred to the urology outpatient clinic. On digital rectal examination, his prostate is enlarged and the serum prostate specific antigen (PSA) level is elevated. What is the most likely finding on IVU?

A A beaded appearance of the distal urethra

B A smooth rounded filling defect at the dome of the bladder

C J-shaped ('fish-hook') appearance of the distal ureters

D Inferior displacement of the ureters by the prostate

E Narrowing of the distal ureters

Answer on page 275

QUESTION 79

A 28-year-old woman has a strong family history of breast cancer and is referred for an MRI examination of the breasts. Regarding MRI of the breast, which one of the following statements is correct?

A Breast MRI should be performed during the middle of the menstrual cycle to improve sensitivity.

B Malignant lesions tend to show poor enhancement following intravenous contrast, compared with surrounding breast tissue.

C MRI has a high sensitivity and specificity for the detection of invasive breast cancer.

D Post radiotherapy, abnormal enhancement patterns return to normal within 3–6 months.

E The patient is imaged in a supine position with the breasts placed in a dedicated breast coil to improve signal to noise ratio.

Answer on page 276

QUESTION 80

Which one of the following statements best describes the characteristic radiological features of retroperitoneal fibrosis?

A A plaque-like mass that encases the aorta and displaces it laterally, most commonly to the left

B A plaque-like mass that displaces the kidneys and ureters laterally at the L1–2 level

C A plaque-like mass that displaces the aorta and iliac arteries anteriorly

D A plaque-like mass that narrows and displaces the ureters laterally at the L4–5 level

E A plaque-like mass that narrows and medially displaces the ureters at the L4–5 level

Answer on page 276

Genitourinary, Adrenal, Obstetric & Gynaecology and Breast

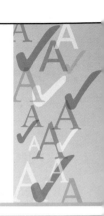

ANSWERS

QUESTION 1

ANSWER: D

The clinical history and ultrasound appearances are highly suggestive of testicular seminoma.

Reference: *Grainger & Allison's* 5e, pp 939–941.

QUESTION 2

ANSWER: C

MRI is the most accurate imaging modality to differentiate T3a from T3b carcinoma. On T2w sequences, an uninterrupted low signal intensity bladder wall seen between the tumour and the surrounding fat excludes extension into the perivesical fat, limiting the tumour to stage T3a.

Reference: *Grainger & Allison's* 5e, pp 892–893.

QUESTION 3

ANSWER: D

The *Clinical Radiology* pictorial review on the ultrasound appearances of testicular epidermoid cysts provides an excellent supplement to *G&A*.

References: *Grainger & Allison's* 5e, pp 940–941.
Atchley JTM, Dewbury KC. Ultrasound appearances of testicular epidermoid cysts: pictorial review. *Clin Radiol* 2000;55(7):493–502.

QUESTION 4

ANSWER: B

The section on testicular torsion within the comprehensive review by Fütterer et al provides useful additional information.

References: *Grainger & Allison's* 5e, p 946.
Fütterer JJ, Heijmink SW, Spermon JR. Imaging the male reproductive tract: current trends and future directions. *Radiol Clin North Am* 2008;46(1):133–147.

QUESTION 5

ANSWER: E

In the early phase of acute orchitis, there is oedema of the testis leading to swelling and diffuse low reflectivity on ultrasound. The ultrasound appearances then evolve to increasingly well-defined areas of patchy low reflectivity. Colour Doppler flow is typically increased within these areas of low reflectivity.

Reference: Cook JL, Dewbury K. The changes seen on high-resolution ultrasound in orchitis. *Clin Rad* 2000;55:13–18.

QUESTION 6

ANSWER: A

Reference: *Grainger & Allison's* 5e, p 939.

QUESTION 7

ANSWER: E

Diastolic flow reversal in the renal arcuate arteries on spectral Doppler ultrasound is a feature of renal vein thrombosis. Acute tubular necrosis (ATN) and acute rejection are difficult to distinguish on a single Doppler examination because they both cause an increase in the resistive index (> 0.8). Renal artery stenosis does not cause diastolic flow reversal and classically produces a slow rising *parvus et tardus* waveform. An arteriovenous fistula is usually the result of renal biopsies and presents as an area of turbulent high flow within the renal parenchyma.

Reference: Baxter GM. Ultrasound of renal transplantation. *Clin Radiol* 2001;56 (10):802–818.

QUESTION 8

ANSWER: E

MCKD is unilateral; if bilateral it is not compatible with life.

Reference: *Grainger & Allison's* 5e, pp 1555–1558 (Table 66.4 provides a concise summary).

QUESTION 9

ANSWER: D

In papillary necrosis, there is no focal cortical loss, despite papillary/calyceal abnormalities.

Reference: *Grainger & Allison's* 5e, pp 836–837.

QUESTION 10

ANSWER: A

Reference: *Grainger & Allison's* 5e, pp 835–836.

QUESTION 11

ANSWER: E

Xanthogranulomatous pyelonephritis (XGP) is a rare form of low-grade chronic renal infection, characterised by progressive destruction of the renal parenchyma. The histological hallmark is replacement of the renal parenchyma by lipid-laden foamy histiocytes. Women are predominantly affected (in a 3:1 ratio), usually in mid-life (50–60 years) and after a long history of recurrent urinary tract infection or urinary stones. Involvement of both kidneys is exceedingly rare. XGP is diffuse in 90% of cases, but focal XGP can simulate a renal tumour.

References: *Grainger & Allison's* 5e, p 839.
Loffroy R, Guiu B, Watfa J, et al. Xanthogranulomatous pyelonephritis in adults: clinical and radiological findings in diffuse and focal forms. *Clin Radiol* 2007;62(9):884–890.

QUESTION 12

ANSWER: C

Puncture of posterior calyces in the mid- and lower poles is optimal. Upper pole puncture increases the risk of pneumothorax whilst direct puncture of the pelvis increases the risk of major vascular injury and persistent urinary leak. If the renal pelvis is inadvertently punctured with the guidewire, once adequate drainage is obtained, this usually settles with observation.

Reference: Kessel & Robertson. *Interventional Radiology: A Survival Guide*, 2nd edition (Edinburgh: Churchill Livingstone, 2005).

QUESTION 13

ANSWER: C

Reference: *Grainger & Allison's* 5e, pp 878–879.

QUESTION 14

ANSWER: C

Reference: *Grainger & Allison's* 5e, pp 837–839.

QUESTION 15

ANSWER: D

Reference: *Grainger & Allison's* 5e, pp 819–820.

QUESTION 16

ANSWER: C

Reference: *Grainger & Allison's* 5e, pp 843–844 (Figure 39.15 provides a clear summary of the findings).

QUESTION 17

ANSWER: D

Reference: *Grainger & Allison's* 5e, p 849.

QUESTION 18

ANSWER: A

The anterior pararenal space lies between the posterior parietal peritoneum anteriorly and Gerota's fascia posteriorly. This space is only partially closed; medially by fusion of the fascial planes along the aorta and IVC and laterally by the lateroconal fascia.

Reference: *Grainger & Allison's* 5e, pp 817–819.

QUESTION 19

ANSWER: B

The presence of gas within a lesion is virtually diagnostic of an abscess but very rarely seen. Immunocompromised patients and those with diabetes are more prone to renal abscess.

Reference: *Grainger & Allison's* 5e, pp 861–862.

QUESTION 20

ANSWER: B

Reference: *Grainger & Allison's* 5e, pp 866–867.

QUESTION 21

ANSWER: A

Ostial and proximal lesions are usually due to atherosclerotic disease. Ostial stenoses are due to aortic wall atheroma and are prone to elastic recoil; therefore they have poor results with angioplasty alone. As a result, many radiologists will opt for angioplasty and primary stenting in patients with ostial stenoses. Fibromuscular dysplasia typically affects the mid-distal renal artery and responds well to angioplasty alone.

Reference: Kessel & Robertson, *Interventional Radiology: A Survival Guide*.

QUESTION 22

ANSWER: A

References: *Grainger & Allison's* 5e, pp 1219, 1227–1229.
Barwick TD, Rockall AG, Barton DP, et al. Imaging of endometrial carcinoma. *Clin Radiol* 2006;61:545–555.

QUESTION 23

ANSWER: E

CMN is defined as an increase in serum creatinine by more than 25% or by 44µmol/L above baseline within 3 days of contrast administration. Prophylactic haemodialysis does not reduce the incidence of CMN but haemofiltration does.

Reference: Morcos SK. Prevention of contrast media nephrotoxicity—the story so far. *Clin Radiol* 2004;59:381–389.

QUESTION 24

ANSWER: A

The 10-HU threshold is now the standard by which radiologists differentiate lipid-rich adenomas from most other adrenal lesions on unenhanced CT. The presence of substantial amounts of intracellular fat is critical in making the specific diagnosis of adenoma. Up to 30% of adenomas, however, do not have abundant intracellular fat and, thus, show attenuation values greater than 10 HU on unenhanced CT. Lesions above 10 HU on an unenhanced CT are considered indeterminate and other investigations may be required.

Reference: Blake MA, Holalkere N, Boland GW. Imaging techniques for adrenal lesion characterization. *Radiol Clin North Am* 2008;46:65–78.

QUESTION 25

ANSWER: A

Stage T3 implies tumour extension through the prostate capsule with/without invasion of the seminal vesicles.

Reference: *Grainger & Allison's* 5e, pp 904–907.

QUESTION 26

ANSWER: D

Ovarian fibromas have characteristic low signal on both T1w and T2w sequences, due to the presence of densely packed connective tissue.

References: *Grainger & Allison's* 5e, p 1236.
Oh SN, Rha SE, Byun JY, et al. MRI features of ovarian fibromas: emphasis on their relationship to the ovary. *Clin Radiol* 2008;63(5):529–535.

QUESTION 27

ANSWER: E

Malignant lesions have abnormally high vascular density leading to slower flow and increased microvascular permeability. This translates to longer transit times for intravenous contrast within malignant adrenal lesions, compared with simple adenomas.

Reference: Blake MA, Holalkere N, Boland GW. Imaging techniques for adrenal lesion characterization. *Radiol Clin North Am* 2008;46:65–78.

QUESTION 28

ANSWER: D

Almost all patients complain of pain/discomfort afterwards and up to 80% will experience either haematuria or haematospermia. Perirectal bleeding (up to 37%), infection, vasovagal attack, urinary retention and epididymitis are other recognised complications. Pneumoperitoneum should not occur because the prostate lies well below the peritoneal reflection.

Reference: Uppot RN, Gervais DA, Mueller PR. Interventional uroradiology. *Radiol Clin North Am* 2008;46:45–64.

QUESTION 29

ANSWER: E

ATN is an early complication in cadaveric allografts and frequently resolves spontaneously in 1–3 weeks. The radionuclide imaging findings of ATN are of preserved perfusion but poor renal function and urine excretion. In acute rejection however, there is both impaired renal function and reduced perfusion on radionuclide imaging.

Reference: He W, Fischman AJ. Nuclear imaging in the genitourinary tract: recent advances and future directions. *Radiol Clin North Am* 2008;46:25–43.

QUESTION 30

ANSWER: A

Phaeochromocytomas are hyperintense on T2w sequences and iso- or hypointense to the liver on T1w sequences.

Reference: Torreggiani WC, Keogh C, Al-Ismail K, et al. Von Hippel-Lindau disease: a radiological essay. *Clin Radiol* 2002;57:670–680.

QUESTION 31

ANSWER: A

Reference: *Grainger & Allison's* 5e, p 921.

QUESTION 32

ANSWER: B

In the setting of a haemodynamically stable patient with a history of major blunt trauma, CT is the most appropriate imaging investigation.

Reference: *Grainger & Allison's* 5e, p 920 (Table 43.1).

QUESTION 33

ANSWER: D

Ureteric injury associated with blunt trauma typically occurs at the pelviureteric junction. Hyperextension with overstretching of the ureter or compression of the ureter against the lumbar transverse processes is the likely mechanism.

Reference: *Grainger & Allison's* 5e, p 928.

QUESTION 34

ANSWER: A

Reference: *Grainger & Allison's* 5e, p 932.

QUESTION 35

ANSWER: A

A deep renal laceration that extends into the collecting system is indicative of a grade 4 injury.

Reference: *Grainger & Allison's* 5e, pp 919–928.

QUESTION 36

ANSWER: E

Reference: *Grainger & Allison's* 5e, p 914.

QUESTION 37

ANSWER: A

A parapelvic cyst is located near the renal hilum, does not communicate with the renal pelvis (unlike calyceal diverticula) and therefore does not opacify during IVU. It compresses the pelvis and may cause hydronephrosis.

Reference: Chapman S, Nakielny R. *Aids to Radiological Differential Diagnosis*, 5th edition (Edinburgh: Saunders, 2003), pp 203–204.

QUESTION 38

ANSWER: C

Angiomyolipomas appear high signal on both T1w and T2w sequences due to their high fat content.

Reference: Chapman & Nakielny, *Aids to Radiological Differential Diagnosis*, pp 205, 207.

QUESTION 39

ANSWER: C

In medullary sponge kidney the kidneys contain numerous medullary cysts which communicate with the tubules and therefore opacify during excretion urography. The cysts contain small calculi giving a 'bunch of grapes appearance'.

References: *Grainger & Allison's* 5e, p 882.
Chapman & Nakielny, *Aids to Radiological Differential Diagnosis*, pp 201–202.

QUESTION 40

ANSWER: B

Theca lutein cysts contain straw-coloured fluid which is low signal on T1w and high signal on T2w images.

Reference: *Grainger & Allison's* 5e, pp 1232–1236.

QUESTION 41

ANSWER: B

Reference: *Grainger & Allison's* 5e, p 914.

QUESTION 42

ANSWER: C

Reference: Chapman & Nakielny, *Aids to Radiological Differential Diagnosis*, p 242.

QUESTION 43

ANSWER: E

Large lesions can extend into and engulf the perinephric fat, and can therefore be mistaken for angiomyolipomas (due to fat content).

Reference: *Grainger & Allison's* 5e, pp 863–864.

QUESTION 44

ANSWER: A

Reference: *Grainger & Allison's* 5e, p 1224.

QUESTION 45

ANSWER: A

Reference: *Grainger & Allison's* 5e, p 1225.

QUESTION 46

ANSWER: B

Fibroadenomas may become calcified, particularly after menopause. Classically the calcifications have a coarse 'popcorn' appearance; however, they may also appear small and punctate. An oil cyst typically demonstrates eggshell calcification and is the result of fat necrosis.

Reference: *Grainger & Allison's* 5e, pp 1180–1181.

QUESTION 47

ANSWER: D

Angiomyolipomas are benign, fat-containing lesions which do not enhance by more than 15 HU and contain low attenuation (−15 to −20HU) fatty areas. Postcontrast enhancement of greater than 20 HU of a solid renal mass is highly suggestive of malignancy.

Reference: *Grainger & Allison's* 5e, p 864.

QUESTION 48

ANSWER: E

Reference: *Grainger & Allison's* 5e, p 1228.

QUESTION 49

ANSWER: B

Reference: *Grainger & Allison's* 5e, p 1194.

QUESTION 50

ANSWER: B

Reference: *Grainger & Allison's* 5e, p 834.

QUESTION 51

ANSWER: A

Mechanical obstruction is associated with elevation of the RI.

Reference: *Grainger & Allison's* 5e, p 872.

QUESTION 52

ANSWER: C

On T2w sequences, the normal bladder wall is of low signal intensity compared with high signal urine. Chemical shift artefact—which in this case is due to the difference in resonant frequencies of the hydrogen nuclei in fat and urine—appears as a dark band on one side wall and a bright band on the opposing wall.

Reference: *Grainger & Allison's* 5e, p 886.

QUESTION 53

ANSWER: B

Reference: *Grainger & Allison's* 5e, pp 871–872 (Table 41.1 provides a concise summary).

QUESTION 54

ANSWER: B

On ultrasound, breast carcinomas are generally ill-defined, hypoechoic masses which can have a surrounding echogenic halo. They also tend to have larger anterior-to-posterior than transverse diameter.

Reference: *Grainger & Allison's* 5e, p 1184.

QUESTION 55

ANSWER: D

Reference: *Grainger & Allison's* 5e, p 819.

QUESTION 56

ANSWER: D

Reference: *Grainger & Allison's* 5e, pp 887–888.

QUESTION 57

ANSWER: D

On dynamic contrast-enhanced MRI, bladder cancer shows earlier enhancement than post-biopsy/surgical tissue and is therefore helpful in distinguishing between bladder cancer and post biopsy change.

Reference: *Grainger & Allison's* 5e, p 893.

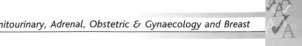

QUESTION 58

ANSWER: C

To provide magnification views, a focal spot of 0.1 mm should be used (smaller than the 0.3 mm focal spot used for standard mammographic projections) with an air gap of 15–30 cm. Options D & E are correct regarding mammography in general and hold true for both standard and magnification views.

References: *Grainger & Allison's* 5e, pp 1173–1175.
Farr RJ, Allisy-Roberts PJ. *Physics for Medical Imaging* (Baillière Tindall, 1996), p 76.

QUESTION 59

ANSWER: C

Malakoplakia is a benign, inflammatory condition that predominantly affects the bladder and lower urinary tract.

Reference: *Grainger & Allison's* 5e, pp 862, 888.

QUESTION 60

ANSWER: B

Seventy per cent of prostate cancers arise from the peripheral zone.

Reference: *Grainger & Allison's* 5e, p 903.

QUESTION 61

ANSWER: D

Reference: *Grainger & Allison's* 5e, p 1174.

QUESTION 62

ANSWER: C

This is the typical description of a Mullerian duct cyst. A seminal vesicle cyst is an important differential; however, they are not usually seen in the midline.

Reference: *Grainger & Allison's* 5e, p 900.

QUESTION 63

ANSWER: D

Zonal anatomy of the prostate is best demonstrated on T2w sequences.

Reference: *Grainger & Allison's* 5e, p 899.

QUESTION 64

ANSWER: B

The central zone atrophies with age whilst the transitional zone enlarges by developing benign prostatic hypertrophy (BPH).

Reference: *Grainger & Allison's* 5e, p 897.

QUESTION 65

ANSWER: B

Prostatic abscess is a localised process which usually begins in the peripheral zone of the gland but may spread to other areas. The incidence is increased in diabetic or immunocompromised patients.

Reference: *Grainger & Allison's* 5e, pp 900–901.

QUESTION 66

ANSWER: D

Invasion of the seminal vesicles is demonstrated by an increase in size of the gland, decrease in signal intensity on T2w images and obliteration of the angle between the seminal vesicles and the posterior bladder wall.

Reference: *Grainger & Allison's* 5e, p 893.

QUESTION 67

ANSWER: E

Postcontrast STIR sequences are pointless as gadolinium shortens T1 and STIR removes signal from tissue with a short T1.

Reference: *Grainger & Allison's* 5e, pp 892–893.

QUESTION 68

ANSWER: E

Women between the ages of 50 and 70 are invited for screening every 3 years. Women over 70 are encouraged to attend by self-referral but are not invited.

Reference: *Grainger & Allison's* 5e, pp 1191–1195.

QUESTION 69

ANSWER: B

In polycystic ovarian syndrome, the ovaries are enlarged with an echogenic central stroma and more than ten peripherally placed cysts (each less than 9 mm in diameter). Option A describes ovarian hyperstimulation syndrome.

Reference: *Grainger & Allison's* 5e, pp 1202, 1233.

QUESTION 70

ANSWER: E

Uric acid stones are not visible on plain radiographs but are seen on CT.

Reference: *Grainger & Allison's* 5e, p 879.

QUESTION 71

ANSWER: E

The central zone atrophies with age while the transitional zone increases in size as it develops BPH. Peripheral zone enlargement is not a feature of BPH.

Reference: *Grainger & Allison's* 5e, pp 897–898.

QUESTION 72

ANSWER: E

Intraperitoneal bladder rupture tends to be due to a tear at the bladder dome. Cystography shows accumulation of contrast at the dome with extravasation laterally outlining bowel loops.

Reference: *Grainger & Allison's* 5e, pp 889–890.

QUESTION 73

ANSWER: D

Reference: *Grainger & Allison's* 5e, p 1238.

QUESTION 74

ANSWER: B

Reference: *Grainger & Allison's* 5e, p 1203 (Figure 53.2).

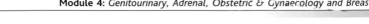

QUESTION 75

ANSWER: D

On CT, as a general rule, the prostate is not considered to be enlarged if an image obtained 1 cm above the symphysis does not include the prostate. Unequivocal enlargement of the prostate is diagnosed if the prostate is seen in images 2–3 cm or more above the symphysis pubis.

Reference: *Grainger & Allison's* 5e, pp 902–903.

QUESTION 76

ANSWER: B

In schistosomiasis, the ureters become grossly dilated and tortuous and may have multiple filling defects due to either granulomata or ureteritis cystica. The urinary bladder becomes small and fibrosed.

Reference: *Grainger & Allison's* 5e, pp 839, 888.

QUESTION 77

ANSWER: B

Extraperitoneal bladder rupture is more common (50–85%) than either intraperitoneal (15–45%) or mixed intra- and extraperitoneal bladder rupture (0–12%). Extraperitoneal bladder rupture is frequently associated (89–100%) with pelvic fractures.

Reference: *Grainger & Allison's* 5e, pp 889–890.

QUESTION 78

ANSWER: C

When the prostate enlarges, it pushes up into the base of the urinary bladder. As a result the trigone is elevated which pushes up the distal ureters (giving a characteristic 'fish-hook' appearance).

Reference: *Grainger & Allison's* 5e, pp 902–903.

QUESTION 79

ANSWER: D

Malignant breast lesions enhance postcontrast; however, normal hormonally active breast tissue can also enhance, particularly during the middle of the menstrual cycle (6th–17th days). In younger patients it may be helpful to repeat the scan earlier or later in the menstrual cycle to improve specificity.

Reference: *Grainger & Allison's* 5e, pp 1189–1190.

QUESTION 80

ANSWER: E

Reference: *Grainger & Allison's* 5e, p 877.

Paediatrics

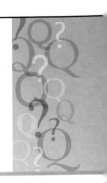

QUESTIONS

QUESTION 1

A 6-month-old child presents to the Emergency Department with a reduced conscious level. There is no history of trauma, but he appears neglected. No physical injury is identified on clinical examination. A CT head is performed. Which one of the following is the most common intracranial finding in nonaccidental injury (NAI)?

  A Hydrocephalus
  B Intracerebral haemorrhage
  C Loss of grey–white matter differentiation
  D Subdural haematoma
  E Subarachnoid haemorrhage

Answer on page 318

QUESTION 2

At a routine 12-week antenatal scan, bowel is seen herniating through an anterior midline abdominal wall defect of the fetus. The umbilical sac measures 25 mm and contains ascites. No other abnormality is detected. The mother's alpha fetal protein is raised. Which one of the following statements is true regarding congenital abdominal wall defects?

A Approximately half of all omphalocoeles are associated with other chromosomal abnormalities.

B If the hernia contains liver, gastroschisis is the most likely diagnosis.

C In gastroschisis, the defect is in the midline.

D In greater than 50% of omphalocoele patients there is associated intestinal atresia.

E In omphalocoele the bowel wall appears thickened.

Answer on page 318

QUESTION 3

A 3-day-old neonate becomes dyspnoeic and requires a chest radiograph. Which one of the following statements will be true regarding the chest radiograph in this neonate?

A The ribs are more vertical than those in an older child's radiograph.

B A normal thymus may compress mediastinal structures.

C The cardiothoracic ratio (CTR) may be as large as 80%.

D The thymus may involute if the child is given steroid treatment.

E The sternum is fully ossified.

Answer on page 318

QUESTION 4

A 7-year-old boy has fallen on an outstretched hand and complains of a painful right elbow. When reviewing the radiographs for evidence of bony injury, which one of the following statements is true?

A A posterior fat pad may be a normal finding on a flexed lateral view.

B An anterior fat pad is always abnormal.

C The line from the anterior cortex of the humerus should pass through the anterior third of the capitellum.

D The medial condyle epiphysis is not normally present on a radiograph at 7 years of age.

E The radiocapitellar line should intersect on all views.

Answer on page 319

QUESTION 5

A baby undergoes an upper GI study which confirms oesophageal atresia with an associated tracheo-oesophageal fistula. Regarding the fistula which of the following statements are true?

A Oesophageal atresia and an H-type fistula is the commonest association.

B On an abdominal radiograph, a gasless abdomen is seen with an H-type fistula.

C The atretic segment is usually located between the middle and distal thirds of the oesophagus.

D The TOF is best demonstrated in the supine position, while injecting contrast.

E The TOF is usually found above the level of the carina.

Answer on page 319

QUESTION 6

A mother is concerned about the shape of her 2-year-old son's head. The GP agrees that it appears elongated and he is referred for skull radiographs and a CT head to look for evidence of craniosynostosis. Which one of the following statements is true regarding congenital skull abnormalities?

A Apert's syndrome is associated with sagittal synostosis.

B Brachycephaly is associated with a higher incidence of neurological abnormalities compared with scaphocephaly.

C Crouzon syndrome affects only the coronal sutures.

D Sagittal synostosis is often seen with hydrocephalus.

E Synostosis of the lamboid suture is more common than the sagittal suture.

Answer on page 319

QUESTION 7

A 2-year-old boy presents with repeated urinary tract infections. Which one of the following investigations would be the most appropriate investigation?

A Intravenous urogram at 6 weeks

B Micturating cystogram at 6 weeks

C Tc-99m DMSA renal scintigraphy at 4 months

D Tc-99m DTPA indirect cystography at 4 months

E An ultrasound at 4 months

Answer on page 319

QUESTION 8

A 5-year-old boy of African origin presents with a 2-week history of a painful right shoulder. He has long-standing lower back pain. His temperature is 38°C. Past medical history is limited, but he has been unwell for some time. Radiographs of his right shoulder and thoracic spine show avascular necrosis of the humeral head and several H-shaped vertebrae. What is the most likely diagnosis?

A Diabetes

B Hypoparathyroidism

C Lead poisoning

D Sickle cell anaemia

E Thalassaemia

Answer on page 320

QUESTION 9

A newborn delivered by caesarean section shows signs of respiratory distress soon after birth. A chest radiograph is performed. Which one of the following features favours the diagnosis of transient tachypnoea of the newborn (TTN)?

A A ground glass appearance throughout both lungs

B Hyper inflated lungs

C Loss of lung volume

D Radiographic resolution after 2 weeks

E The presence of a pleural effusion

Answer on page 320

QUESTION 10

An 18-month-old infant presents with failure to thrive and anorexia. On examination an upper abdominal mass is palpable. Blood tests reveal an iron deficiency anaemia and a raised alpha fetal protein. The clinicians wish to exclude a hepatoblastoma. When imaging this child, which one of the following statements holds true?

A Angiography should be performed to establish vascular anatomy.

B Calcification will be seen on a plain abdominal radiograph in 5–10% of cases.

C Following contrast administration, there is centripetal and heterogeneous enhancement on CT.

D Hepatoblastoma demonstrates increased activity during the delayed phase of Tc-99m sulphur colloid scintigraphy.

E Ultrasound characteristically demonstrates a focal echogenic mass.

Answer on page 320

QUESTION 11

A 4-week-old male neonate presents with nonbilious vomiting and a hypochloraemic alkalosis. Hypertrophic pyloric stenosis is suspected and an ultrasound is performed. Which one of the following ultrasound findings would confirm the diagnosis?

A A pylorus that does not open

B Pyloric canal length of greater than 11 mm

C Pyloric muscle wall thickness of 1 mm

D Reduced gastric peristalsis

E Transverse pyloric diameter of greater than 11 mm

Answer on page 320

QUESTION 12

A 4-year-old child presents with upper back pain. General examination reveals hepatomegaly and blood tests demonstrate an iron deficiency anaemia. The child's chest radiograph demonstrates an abnormal mediastinal contour and subsequent CT confirms an 8-cm posterior mediastinal mass which contains calcification. The lungs are clear. Which one of the following is most likely the diagnosis?

A Extramedullary haemopoiesis
B Lymphoma
C Neuroblastoma
D Neurofibroma
E Teratoma

Answer on page 321

QUESTION 13

On an antenatal ultrasound of a male fetus, bilateral hydronephrosis was identified. A subsequent ultrasound demonstrates worsening hydronephrosis with a full bladder and reduced volume of amniotic fluid. As a result labour is induced early. Which one of the following postnatal investigations will provide a definitive diagnosis?

A A repeat postnatal ultrasound
B Cystography
C DMSA renal scintigraphy
D Micturating cystourethrography
E Tc-99m MAG scintigram

Answer on page 321

QUESTION 14

A 6-month-old child with a palpable abdominal mass is initially investigated
with an ultrasound, revealing a mixed echogenic mass in the left kidney.
A subsequent CT demonstrates a large mass within the left kidney which has a
moderately enhancing component. Which one of the following would be
the most likely diagnosis?

A Angiomyolipoma

B Lymphoma

C Nephroblastomatosis

D Neuroblastoma

E Wilms' tumour

Answer on page 321

QUESTION 15

A 3-month-old infant presents with a history of failure to thrive.
On examination, the infant is tachypnoeic with no clinical evidence of central
or peripheral cyanosis. A chest radiograph shows enlarged central and
peripheral pulmonary vessels throughout both lungs. Which one of the
following is a potential diagnosis?

A Pulmonary stenosis

B Tetralogy of Fallot

C Total anomalous pulmonary venous return

D Tricuspid atresia

E Ventricular septal defect (VSD)

Answer on page 321

QUESTION 16

Interstitial lung disease is suspected in a 3-year-old child who has a long history of breathlessness on exertion. A chest radiograph reveals interstitial change at the lung bases. The clinical symptoms are more severe than the radiographic changes appear to suggest and a diagnosis is yet to be established. Which one of the following would be the next appropriate investigation?

A Bronchoscopy

B Contrast-enhanced chest CT

C HRCT

D MRI

E Noncontrast chest CT

Answer on page 321

QUESTION 17

A 5-year-old boy is involved in a traffic accident and is complaining of neck pain. Which of the following statements is true regarding the cervical spine radiograph?

A Subluxation of up to 7 mm of C2 anteriorly on C3 is normal.

B Subluxation of up to 3 mm of C2 posteriorly on C3 is normal.

C The distance between the anterior arch of C1 and the dens can be up to 5 mm.

D The soft tissues anterior to C2 must be no wider than 1/4 of the width of the C2 vertebral body.

E The soft tissues anterior to C6 must be no wider than 1/2 of the width of the C6 vertebral body.

Answer on page 322

QUESTION 18

A 2-year-old-year-old child of Mediterranean origin presents for the first time with severe iron deficiency anaemia. Blood tests reveal he is a beta thalassaemia major carrier. A skeletal survey is performed. Which of the following is a recognised radiographic finding in beta thalassaemia?

A Enlargement of the frontal sinuses

B Erlenmeyer flask deformity of the femora

C Long bone diaphyseal periosteal new bone formation

D Lucent metaphyseal bands

E Medial displacement of the orbits

Answer on page 322

QUESTION 19

A 5-year-old presents with a 2-month history of a painful right knee.
On radiograph, there is a poorly defined lytic lesion in the distal femoral metaphysis, with an associated sunburst type periosteal reaction. An MRI is performed to classify this lesion further. Which one of the following imaging protocols would you choose?

A CT chest, abdomen and pelvis, with MRI T1w and T2w axial and coronal sequences of the femur

B CT chest, with MRI T1w and T2w axial, sagittal, coronal sequences of the femur

C Isotope bone scan, CT abdomen with MRI T1w and T2w sagittal, coronal, axial sequences of the femur

D Isotope bone scan, CT chest with MRI T1w and T2w sagittal, axial, coronal sequences of the femur

E MRI T1w and T2w axial, sagittal and coronal sequences of the femur

Answer on page 322

QUESTION 20

A 2-week-old baby presents with poor feeding and bilious vomiting.
Physical examination is unremarkable. Malrotation is suspected and an upper
GI contrast study is requested. What specific radiological findings would
confirm the diagnosis?

A 'Corkscrewing' of the duodenum and jejunum

B On the supine radiograph the D-J flexure lies to the left of the midline.

C On a lateral view the D-J flexure is posterior.

D On the supine radiograph the D-J flexure lies above the duodenal bulb.

E The caecal pole position is abnormal.

Answer on page 322

QUESTION 21

A neonate presents at 24 hours old with vomiting, abdominal distension
and failure to pass meconium. A series of investigations are performed.
Which of the following would be in keeping with a diagnosis of meconium
ileus?

A A contrast enema showing a dilated terminal ileum

B A contrast enema showing pellets of meconium within the terminal
ileum

C A contrast study showing narrow loops of proximal ileum

D A plain abdominal radiograph with a soap bubble appearance within the
left iliac fossa

E An ultrasound showing echo poor bowel loops

Answer on page 323

QUESTION 22

A 5-year-old child presents with pyrexia and weight loss. The urine cultures reveal *Proteus mirabilis*. An ultrasound demonstrates an enlarged kidney, consistent with an inflammatory mass. Xanthogranulomatous pyelonephritis is considered. Which one of the following statements is true regarding the imaging findings of this condition?

A Calcification is rarely seen on CT.

B Hot spots are seen on a Tc-99m DMSA scan.

C On MRI the necrotic areas tend to be high signal on T2w images with medium signal intensity on T1w images.

D Perinephric extension is unusual on both CT and MRI.

E The infected cavities enhance avidly with intravenous contrast on CT.

Answer on page 323

QUESTION 23

Following a recent viral illness, a 5-year-old girl presents with a fluctuating conscious level, seizures and left leg weakness. She is apyrexial and does not have a rash. An MRI is performed. This shows bilateral areas of increased T2 signal in the subcortical white matter and cerebellum and deep grey matter. Which one of the following is the most likely diagnosis?

A Acute disseminated encephalomyelitis (ADEM)

B Bacterial meningitis

C Multiple sclerosis

D Venous sinus thrombosis

E Viral encephalitis

Answer on page 323

QUESTION 24

A 3-day-old neonate demonstrates signs of respiratory distress. A chest radiograph demonstrates a right pleural effusion. Which of the following is the commonest cause?

A Chylothorax
B Hydrops fetalis
C Meconium aspiration syndrome
D Pulmonary haemorrhage
E Respiratory distress syndrome

Answer on page 323

QUESTION 25

An infant born at 38 weeks' gestation has suffered hypoxic birth trauma. In which of the following locations are you most likely to see abnormalities on MRI?

A Cerebellar peduncles
B Midbrain
C Periventricular region
D Subcortical white matter of the frontal cortex
E Thalami

Answer on page 324

QUESTION 26

A 6-month-old infant presents with jaundice, upper abdominal discomfort and an abdominal mass. An ultrasound is performed. Which of the following findings would suggest a choledochal cyst?

A A gradual transition between dilated and nondilated portions

B An absent gallbladder

C Fusiform dilatation of the pancreatic duct

D Multiple low reflective areas with a central focus of high reflectivity in the liver

E Proximal intrahepatic duct saccular dilatation

Answer on page 324

QUESTION 27

An 8-month-old child who was previously well presents with vomiting and an altered conscious level. A CT head reveals significant hydrocephalus with a hyperdense mass. An MRI is arranged and reveals a lobulated mass adjacent to the trigone of a lateral ventricle. This lesion yields low signal on both T1w and T2w sequences with avid enhancement postcontrast. Which one of the following is the most likely diagnosis?

A Choroid plexus tumour

B Craniopharyngioma

C Ependymoma

D Lymphoma

E Meningioma

Answer on page 324

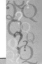

QUESTION 28

A 13-year-old girl presents with a 3-month history of nonspecific neck ache with muscle spasm. A radiograph of her cervical spine reveals a 3-cm lucent lesion with a sclerotic rim in the posterior elements of C4. There is minimal periosteal reaction. Bone scintigraphy demonstrates a region of intense uptake correlating with the radiographic findings. On MRI, the lesion yields low signal on T1w and medium to high signal on T2w sequences, as well as mild bone marrow oedema. Which one of the following is the most likely diagnosis?

A Aneurysmal bone cyst (ABC)

B Nonossifying fibroma (NOF)

C Osteoid osteoma

D Osteoblastoma

E Osteosarcoma

Answer on page 324

QUESTION 29

Immediately following delivery, a neonate experiences respiratory difficulties. On examination the trachea is deviated to the left, and there is reduced air entry on the right. A chest radiograph confirms mediastinal deviation to the left with an opaque right hemithorax. A NG tube is passed and a further chest radiograph is performed. This demonstrates that the stomach lies within the chest cavity. Which one of the following best describes the most common site and size of a congenital diaphragmatic hernia?

A Anterior, small and left sided

B Anterior, small and right sided

C Posterior, large and left sided

D Posterior, large and right sided

E Posterior, small and right sided

Answer on page 325

QUESTION 30

A 5-year-old boy who had a coarctation of his aorta repaired 12 months ago requires follow-up. Which of the following imaging modalities is the gold standard?

   A Conventional angiography
   B CT
   C Echocardiogram
   D MRI
   E Plain radiograph

Answer on page 325

QUESTION 31

A neonate presents with an abdominal mass. An abdominal radiograph reveals normal bowel gas pattern with no calcification. Ultrasound demonstrates a cystic mass in the left flank. Which one of the following conditions is most likely in this neonate?

   A Hydronephrosis
   B Infantile polycystic kidney
   C Mesonephric nephroma
   D Multicystic dysplastic kidney
   E Wilms' tumour

Answer on page 325

QUESTION 32

A 6-year-old boy presents with a right-sided limp of a few weeks' duration. He is apyrexial. Which one of the following is the earliest radiographic sign that would support a diagnosis of Perthes' disease of the hip?

A A subchondral lucency

B Fragmentation of the femoral head

C Hip effusion

D Periarticular osteopenia

E Sclerosis of the femoral head

Answer on page 325

QUESTION 33

A 5-year-old child presents with vomiting, lethargy and a persistent headache. A CT head is performed and shows a hyperdense midline posterior fossa mass, abutting the fourth ventricle with associated hydrocephalus. There is significant peritumoral oedema but no calcification, and avid homogeneous enhancement is seen postcontrast. On MRI, the mass yields low signal on T1w and is isointense on T2w sequences. Which one of the following posterior fossa tumours is the most likely diagnosis?

A Cerebellar haemangioblastoma

B Choroid plexus tumour

C Ependymoma

D Medulloblastoma

E Pilocytic astrocytoma

Answer on page 326

QUESTION 34

A screening hip ultrasound was performed on a 4-week-old female with a positive family history of developmental dysplasia of the hip (DDH). Which one of the following measurements would confirm DDH in this child?

A An alpha angle of >60°

B An alpha angle of between 55° and 59°

C A beta angle of <55°

D A beta angle of >77°

E Delayed ossification of the acetabular roof

Answer on page 326

QUESTION 35

A 15-year-old girl with cystic fibrosis (CF) presents with vomiting and colicky abdominal pain. Examination reveals a right-sided abdominal mass and the patient appears dehydrated. Initial blood tests are unremarkable and an abdominal radiograph shows small bowel obstruction with faecal loading. Which one of the following is the most likely diagnosis?

A Appendicitis

B Distal intestinal obstruction

C Gallstones

D Meckel's diverticulum

E None of the above

Answer on page 326

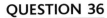

QUESTION 36

A 3-year-old boy presents with 2-month history of a generalised maculopapular rash, a painful swollen left upper arm and nonproductive cough. On examination he appears dyspnoeic and the left humerus is tender but not erythematous. A plain radiograph of the humerus reveals a lucent diaphyseal lesion, with cortical thinning, endosteal scalloping and mild periosteal reaction. A chest radiograph shows reticular nodular shadowing in an upper zone predominance. Which one of the following is the most likely diagnosis?

A Disseminated metastases

B Ewing's sarcoma

C Fibrous dysplasia

D Langerhans cell histiocytosis (LCH)

E Sarcoidosis

Answer on page 326

QUESTION 37

On a routine 20-week antenatal scan, the right fetal kidney contains multiple large cysts varying in size and scattered in a random distribution. No discernible renal tissue is seen. The left kidney appears normal. What is the most likely diagnosis?

A Autosomal recessive polycystic kidney disease

B Medullary sponge kidney

C Multicystic dysplastic kidney

D Multiple simple cysts

E Tuberous sclerosis

Answer on page 327

QUESTION 38

A large posterior fossa cyst is identified during an antenatal ultrasound scan. Following delivery the diagnosis of a Dandy Walker malformation is being considered. In addition to a large posterior fossa cystic mass which one of the following abnormalities would support this diagnosis?

A Agenesis of the septum pellucidum

B Hypoplastic cerebellar vermis

C Inferiorly displaced fourth ventricle

D Myelomeningocoele

E Tectal plate beaking

Answer on page 327

QUESTION 39

A child attends the Medical Physics Department for a Tc-99m DTPA renal isotope study. Which one of the following statements is a justified indication for the scan?

A Assessment of renal scarring

B Establishing divided renal function

C Follow-up of pyelonephritis

D Investigating recurrent urinary tract infections

E Suspected duplex kidney

Answer on page 327

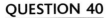

QUESTION 40

A 15-year-old boy presents with a painful right knee which is aggravated by sport. It occasionally swells and locks, but clinical examination does not reveal any ligamentous instability. A plain radiograph appears normal and an MRI is performed and shows evidence of osteochondritis dissecans. Which one of the following statements is true regarding the imaging findings in this condition?

- **A** Associated loose bodies are seen.
- **B** Decreased signal within subchondral bone is seen on proton density MR images.
- **C** MRI is of little use in predicting stability of fractures.
- **D** The lateral condyle is most commonly involved.
- **E** The plain radiograph is always normal.

Answer on page 327

QUESTION 41

A 2-year-old has an elbow radiograph performed following a fall. Which one of the following epiphyses should be visible?

- **A** Capitellum
- **B** Medial epicondyle
- **C** None
- **D** Olecranon
- **E** Radial head

Answer on page 328

QUESTION 42

A 5-year-old child with CF presents with right upper abdominal pain. The full blood count and liver functions blood tests are normal. An abdominal radiograph is also normal. When investigating this patient which one of the following statements is true?

A A CT would be the next line of investigation.

B An ultrasound will only detect liver disease in its late stages.

C Greater than 50% of CF patients have gallstones on ultrasound.

D On ultrasound, the appendix appears larger than normal in CF.

E The incidence of intussusception is not increased in CF.

Answer on page 328

QUESTION 43

It has been decided that a newborn baby requiring respiratory support also requires increased monitoring via arterial and venous umbilical catheters. Radiographs have been taken to confirm their positions. Which of the following statements is true?

A The tip of the arterial line should lie above T6.

B The tip of the arterial line should lie between T10 and L3.

C The tip of the venous line should lie within the liver.

D The tip of the venous line should lie within the superior vena cava (SVC).

E The venous line should pass through the left portal vein.

Answer on page 328

QUESTION 44

A 2-year-old is being investigated for abnormal head growth with serial skull radiographs. Which one of the following statements is true?

A Rickets is a recognised cause of widened sutures.

B Secondary causes of widened cranial sutures are unusual.

C Sickle cell disease is a recognised cause of widened sutures.

D Suture widths of 3 mm for a 2-year-old are considered abnormal.

E Thalassaemia is a recognised cause of widened sutures.

Answer on page 328

QUESTION 45

A 3-month-old baby is brought to the Emergency Department with a reduced conscious level. The history is unclear and inconsistent and NAI is strongly suspected. A CT head is performed. Which one of the following findings would be most suggestive of NAI rather than an alternative diagnosis?

A Hydrocephalus

B Interhemispheric subdural haemorrhage

C Leptomeningeal enhancement

D Linear parietal skull fracture

E Periventricular white matter ischaemia

Answer on page 328

QUESTION 46

On a 20-week antenatal ultrasound, unilateral fetal hydronephrosis is detected. Which one of the following findings would confirm the diagnosis of renal pelvic dilatation (RPD)?

A During the second trimester, the AP renal pelvis measures more than 3 mm.

B During the third trimester, the AP renal pelvis measures greater than 5 mm.

C Megaureters are present.

D The AP renal pelvis measures greater than 25% of the longitudinal length of the kidney.

E The AP renal pelvis measures greater than 50% of the longitudinal length of the kidney.

Answer on page 329

QUESTION 47

A 3-year-old girl presents with a purpuric rash, abdominal pain and blood-stained stools. The ESR is raised. Henoch-Schönlein purpura (HSP) is the clinical diagnosis. Which one of the following statements is true when investigating this child?

A An ultrasound is of little diagnostic use.

B An ultrasound finding of hypoechoic, thickened bowel wall with echogenic areas would be supportive of the clinical diagnosis.

C If an intussusception is seen it is likely to be difficult to reduce.

D Involvement of the GI tract is seen in 10% of patients with HSP.

E The commonest site of GI involvement is the terminal ileum.

Answer on page 329

QUESTION 48

A neonate with an uncomplicated antenatal and birth history has had jaundice for 14 days. On examination he is mildly dehydrated and is referred for investigation of persistent jaundice. When considering the imaging of biliary atresia, which one of the following statements is true?

A Twenty per cent of infants with persistent neonatal jaundice will have biliary atresia or neonatal hepatitis.

B A normal gallbladder which distends with fasting suggests an alternative diagnosis.

C In biliary atresia, cirrhosis is not prevented by biliary decompression.

D In biliary atresia, the liver shows decreased periportal reflectivity on ultrasound.

E Tc-99m sulphur colloid is used to confirm the diagnosis of biliary atresia.

Answer on page 329

QUESTION 49

A 4-year-old child presents with groin pain and haematuria. An ultrasound is performed and suggests crossed fused ectopic kidney. Which one of the following statements is true regarding the anatomy of renal anomalies?

A In crossed fused ectopia, both of the kidneys are abnormally placed.

B In crossed fused ectopia, both ureters enter the bladder in a normal position.

C In crossed fused ectopia, the crossed kidney is fused superiorly to the other.

D The upper poles are fused in a horseshoe kidney.

E The ureters pass posterior to the lower poles in a horseshoe kidney.

Answer on page 329

QUESTION 50

A 5-year-old child presented 1 week ago with bacterial meningitis and is now persistently pyrexial with new onset seizures. An MRI shows frontal leptomeningeal enhancement, with enhancing material within the subdural space. The signal from the subdural space is higher than CSF in both the T1w and T2w images. What is the most likely diagnosis?

A Cerebral abscess
B Cerebritis
C Subdural effusion
D Subdural empyema
E Ventriculitis

Answer on page 330

QUESTION 51

An 11-year-old boy presents with right hip pain. He is apyrexial and the clinicians are concerned that he has a slipped upper femoral epiphysis. Which one of the following would be appropriate first-line imaging?

A AP and frogleg lateral radiographs of the pelvis
B CT with 3D reconstruction of the affected hip joint
C MRI T1w, T2w and proton density fat-saturated images of the right hip
D PA and frogleg lateral radiographs of the pelvis
E Ultrasound of the hip

Answer on page 330

QUESTION 52

A newborn baby is hypoxic immediately following delivery. There is evidence of meconium-stained amniotic fluid. Which one of the following statements is true regarding meconium aspiration syndrome?

A Radiological resolution is usually seen within 48–72 hours.

B Pneumothorax and pneumomediastinum are uncommon complications.

C The chest radiograph typically shows a fine ground glass appearance.

D The chest radiograph typically shows patchy consolidation with areas of hyperinflation.

E The chest radiograph typically shows unilateral abnormalities.

Answer on page 330

QUESTION 53

A 3-month-old infant with Tetralogy of Fallot is awaiting surgery. A preoperative chest radiograph is performed when the child has no concurrent illness. Which one of the following features are you most likely to see?

A Boot-shaped heart

B Enlarged hila

C Pulmonary plethora

D Rib notching

E Splaying of hila

Answer on page 330

QUESTION 54

A neonate who is cyanotic at birth undergoes an echocardiogram. This detects apical displacement of the septal leaves of the tricuspid valve and an apical septal defect. Which one of the following is the most likely diagnosis?

A Bacterial endocarditis

B Ebstein's anomaly

C Eisenmenger's syndrome

D Tetralogy of Fallot

E Tricuspid atresia

Answer on page 330

QUESTION 55

A 1-year-old girl is being investigated for repeated urinary tract infections. She undergoes an ultrasound which shows a left duplex kidney with a dilated upper collecting system and a large left ureterocoele. Which one of the following statements is true?

A Ectopic drainage of the ureter is rarely associated with scarring of the kidney.

B The ureter draining the lower moiety usually enters the bladder as a ureterocoele.

C The ureter draining the upper moiety usually enters the bladder as a ureterocoele.

D The ureter draining the upper moiety is usually affected by reflux.

E When one moiety drains outside the bladder, it is usually the lower pole.

Answer on page 331

QUESTION 56

A 2-week-old septic neonate shows worsening renal function and proteinuria. He is currently being monitored on the paediatric ITU. Seven days after his initial illness, an ultrasound is performed which reveals a unilateral enlarged kidney, with loss of corticomedullary differentiation and reversal of end diastolic arterial flow. Associated adrenal haemorrhage is noted. What is the most likely diagnosis?

A Acute glomerulonephritis

B Acute tubular necrosis

C Renal artery stenosis

D Renal vein thrombosis

E Unilateral obstruction

Answer on page 331

QUESTION 57

An 8-year-old boy presents with a 3-month history of feeling tired and unwell with pain and stiffness in his hips and knees. Blood tests reveal an elevated ESR and a haemoglobin of 9.8 g/dL. Plain radiographs are taken of the symptomatic joints. Which of the following statements is true when considering the diagnosis of juvenile idiopathic arthritis (JIA)?

A A widened intercondylar notch is a recognised finding.

B Ankylosis of carpal bones is unusual.

C Juxta-articular osteoporosis is not seen.

D Narrowing of the joint spaces is seen in the early stages of the disease.

E The hip is the most commonly affected joint.

Answer on page 331

QUESTION 58

The clinical course of a premature neonate is complicated by abdominal distension and diarrhoea. An radiograph is taken to exclude necrotising enterocolitis (NEC). Regarding the potential radiographic findings, which one of the following is true?

A A persistent, solitary dilated loop is an indicator of impending perforation.

B Gaseous distension of large bowel is a late radiological sign.

C Pneumatosis intestinalis is specific to NEC.

D Portal venous gas is seen in more than half of clinical cases.

E The disappearance of portal venous gas indicates recovery.

Answer on page 331

QUESTION 59

You are asked to perform a Gastrografin enema on a baby with confirmed meconium ileus. You are required to set up for the procedure and communicate with the clinicians. Which one of the following statements is correct?

A Full strength Gastrografin is recommended, in order to give the best imaging.

B The enema can only be performed once, after which surgery is the preferred option.

C The success rate in relieving the obstruction is over 90%.

D The risk of perforation during the procedure is around 5%.

E You should proceed quickly, when the baby is poorly hydrated, in order to achieve a quicker result.

Answer on page 331

QUESTION 60

A 6-month-old infant who had a normal clinical examination at birth presents with failure to thrive and cyanotic episodes. Physical examination reveals a left sternal edge murmur. An echocardiogram demonstrates a patent ductus arteriosus (PDA). Which one of the following statements regarding a PDA is true?

A A large PDA typically results in Eisenmenger's syndrome developing during childhood.

B A small PDA can be left untreated.

C It is associated with left isomerism.

D It is seen as part of Tetralogy of Fallot.

E The radiograph of a child with a PDA classically shows pulmonary plethora.

Answer on page 332

QUESTION 61

Primary sagittal synostosis is suspected in a 3-month-old infant and a series of plain skull radiographs are taken. Which one of the following statements is correct?

A Lambdoid and sagittal sutures are examined on the Townes' projection.

B The AP projection is the best view to assess the foramen magnum and the fontanelles.

C The AP projection will only assess lambdoid and metopic sutures.

D The AP projection will only assess the coronal and the sagittal sutures.

E The sagittal and lambdoid sutures are examined on a lateral projection.

Answer on page 332

QUESTION 62

A 3-year-old boy who is otherwise well presents with a 6-month history of generalised back pain. An radiograph of the thoracic spine demonstrates collapse of T11, T12 and L1 vertebral bodies. A skeletal survey is performed which identifies several punched out lesions in the skull, with sclerotic edges. Which one of the following is the most likely diagnosis?

A Fibrous dysplasia

B Gaucher's disease

C Langerhans cell histiocytosis

D Lymphoma

E Metastases

Answer on page 332

QUESTION 63

A 14-day-old neonate is undergoing an ultrasound to investigate jaundice. Which one of the following statements is true regarding normal ultrasound anatomy in a newborn?

A Splenic anomalies are unusual.

B The newborn liver is more reflective than the kidney.

C The umbilical vein drains into the left portal vein.

D The umbilical vein is patent up to the age of 6 weeks.

E The upper limit diameter for a common bile duct in a newborn is 5 mm.

Answer on page 332

QUESTION 64

A 3-year-old child presents with weight loss and an abdominal mass. On the initial ultrasound, a large mass is seen in the region of the right kidney/adrenal. A CT abdomen is arranged. Which one of the following statements is correct when differentiating between a Wilms' tumour and neuroblastoma?

A Neuroblastoma enhances more than the adjacent renal parenchyma.

B Neuroblastoma usually displaces rather than encases vessels.

C Pulmonary metastases are more suggestive of Wilms' tumour.

D Skeletal metastases are more suggestive of Wilms' tumour.

E Wilms' tumour is more likely to contain calcification.

Answer on page 333

QUESTION 65

A 3-year-old boy has intermittent abdominal pain in the peri-umbilical region and bright red blood per rectum. A technetium 99m pertechnetate study is performed for a suspected Meckel's diverticulum. When imaging this child which one of the following statements is true?

A Cimetidine given prior to the examination results in reduced tracer uptake by gastric mucosa.

B In children the study will only detect 20–30% of positive Meckel's diverticula.

C In a positive study, a Meckel's diverticulum is typically seen as a focus of tracer uptake in the left lower quadrant.

D In a positive study, the activity in the Meckel's diverticulum appears at the same time and same intensity as the gastric mucosa.

E Malrotation may produce a false positive.

Answer on page 333

QUESTION 66

A term neonate with an unremarkable antenatal history presents at 48 hours with abdominal distension and failure to pass meconium. After a digital rectal examination, stool is passed and Hirschsprung's disease is being considered as a diagnosis. Which one of the following statements is true regarding the diagnosis of this condition?

A A definitive diagnosis can be made on barium enema alone.

B A pneumoperitoneum is seen on 25% of presenting abdominal radiographs.

C On the abdominal radiograph, an absence of rectal gas is specific to Hirschsprung's.

D On an enema, the aganglionic segment extends to the rectosigmoid junction in 70–80% of cases.

E When performing an enema it is important to inflate the rectal catheter balloon in order to achieve a good seal.

Answer on page 333

QUESTION 67

A 2-year-old child presents to the Emergency Department with a greenstick fracture of the ulna. On the radiograph, there is evidence of an old fracture to the same limb and the history given by the parents is inconsistent. NAI is clinically suspected and a skeletal survey is performed. Which of the following fractures have a high specificity for NAI?

A Fractures of multiple ages

B Fracture of the middle third of the clavicle

C Fracture of the lateral third of the clavicle

D Linear skull fracture

E Spiral humeral fracture

Answer on page 333

QUESTION 68

A 3-year-old boy presents with a short history of shortness of breath. Clinical examination is unremarkable, but on the chest radiograph there are multiple pulmonary nodules suggestive of metastases. Which one of the following tumours would be the most likely source of pulmonary metastases in this child?

A Lymphoma

B Medulloblastoma

C Nephroblastoma (Wilms' tumour)

D Neuroblastoma

E Testicular teratoma

Answer on page 334

QUESTION 69

A 4-year-old child presents with shortness of breath and a fever. The chest radiograph shows a round opacity within the right lower zone. No previous radiographs are available for comparison. Which one of the following statements is true when trying to distinguish pneumonia from a tumour in a child?

A Ill-defined margins make pneumonia more likely.

B Pneumonic changes usually persist for several weeks following treatment.

C Sharp margins are associated with a round pneumonia.

D The absence of an air bronchogram makes tumour more likely.

E An MRI would be the next investigation of choice.

Answer on page 334

QUESTION 70

A 2-year-old infant presents with a history of developmental delay, seizures and subcutaneous lesions. The clinicians suspect tuberous sclerosis. Which one of the following radiological findings are consistent with this diagnosis?

A Calcified subependymal nodules

B Leptomeningeal angiomas

C Multiple meningiomas

D Pilocytic astrocytoma

E Retinoblastoma

Answer on page 334

QUESTION 71

An antenatal ultrasound demonstrated a fetus with shortened limbs and hydrocephalus. Following birth a skeletal survey was performed on the infant to confirm or exclude achondroplasia. Which one of the following is a recognised radiological feature of this condition?

A Anterior scalloping of the vertebral bodies

B Biconcave vertebral bodies

C Flat acetabular roofs

D Large foramen magnum

E Widened interpedicular distance in the lumbar spine

Answer on page 334

QUESTION 72

A 1-day-old neonate presents with bilious vomiting. A plain radiograph demonstrates the 'double bubble' sign of the stomach and duodenal cap and complete duodenal obstruction is suspected. When considering this diagnosis, which one of the following statements is true?

A An upper GI contrast study is required to make the diagnosis.

B Down's syndrome is present in 20–30% of patients with duodenal atresia.

C Duodenal stenosis is more common than atresia.

D The level of obstruction is usually proximal to the ampulla of Vater.

E The plain radiograph should be taken in the erect position.

Answer on page 334

QUESTION 73

An 8-month-old boy presents with colicky abdominal pain and redcurrant jelly stool. An abdominal radiograph is unremarkable, but on ultrasound a midline mass is seen with a typical appearance of an intussusception.
The departmental protocol is to reduce the intussusception using pneumatic hydrostatic reduction. Which one of the following statements is true?

A Free intraperitoneal gas on the abdominal radiograph is a contraindication to barium reduction but not pneumatic reduction.

B Maximum insufflation pressure with pneumatic reduction is 150 mmHg.

C Pneumatic reduction has a radiation dose lower than that of barium reduction.

D The absence of blood flow seen on colour Doppler within the intussusceptum indicates vascular compromise and is a contraindication to radiological reduction.

E The presence of intraperitoneal fluid on the ultrasound is a contraindication to pneumatic hydrostatic reduction.

Answer on page 335

QUESTION 74

A 3-year-old Caucasian boy with chronic renal impairment secondary to nephrotic syndrome presents with a painful left arm following a minor fall. On the initial radiograph there is a midshaft fracture of the ulna. The appearance of the radius and ulna are noted to be abnormal with generalised osteopenia and widening of the distal physes. What is the most likely diagnosis?

A Avascular necrosis

B Gaucher's disease

C Nonaccidental injury

D Rickets

E Scurvy

Answer on page 335

QUESTION 75

A neonate presents in the immediate postnatal period with excessive drooling, choking and cyanosis. Polyhydramnios had been detected on antenatal ultrasound and a diagnosis of oesophageal atresia (OA) is suspected. Which one of the following is the most useful first-line investigation to help exclude or confirm OA?

A Pass a nasogastric tube; if stomach contents are aspirated then no further investigations are required.

B Pass a nasogastric tube, then inject a small amount of air followed by a supine chest radiograph.

C Perform a multiplanar CT chest.

D Perform a PA chest radiograph to confirm a gastric air bubble.

E Perform a positive contrast oesophagram.

Answer on page 335

QUESTION 76

A 12-year-old child with CF has been followed up with annual chest radiographs. Which of the following features is a late radiographic change associated with the disease?

A Bronchial wall thickening

B Cavitations

C Consolidation

D Diffuse interstitial pattern

E Hilar enlargement

Answer on page 335

QUESTION 77

A neonate with a history of worsening cyanosis and respiratory distress has a series of chest radiographs taken. The initial chest radiograph reveals a solid left upper lobe mass and over the course of 3 weeks, this becomes aerated. Progressive mediastinal shift is seen as the mass enlarges. Which one of the following is the most likely diagnosis?

A Bronchopulmonary sequestration

B Congenital cystic adenomatoid malformation (CCAM)

C Congenital diaphragmatic hernia

D Congenital lobar emphysema

E Pneumatocoele secondary to *E. coli* infection

Answer on page 335

QUESTION 78

A 5-year-old child with neurofibromatosis type 1 (NF1) presents with a unilateral painless proptosis and reduced visual acuity. He undergoes both CT and MRI examinations of the orbits and brain. When assessing for an optic nerve glioma, which one of the following statements is true?

A Calcification of the optic tract on CT would suggest an optic nerve glioma.

B Extension of the tumour into the subarachnoid space is recognised.

C On T1w images, optic nerve gliomas yield high signal.

D Optic nerve gliomas are usually nonenhancing.

E The commonest location of an optic pathway glioma is within the optic chiasm.

Answer on page 336

QUESTION 79

A 10-month-old girl is being investigated for delayed motor development. An MRI brain is performed under sedation. Which one of the following statements is correct regarding the MRI appearances of normal brain development in a child of this age?

A Adult appearances of the corpus callosum are not expected.

B It is possible to assess myelination accurately using T1w images alone.

C On T1w images, myelination will have almost reached adult maturity by imaging criteria.

D On T2w images, myelination of the optic radiation is abnormal.

E On T2w images, subcortical white matter myelination is seen extending from the frontal cortex into the parietal and temporal lobes.

Answer on page 336

QUESTION 80

A child with known Langerhans cell histiocytosis (LCH) presents with worsening respiratory symptoms. An HRCT chest is performed. Which one of the following statements is true regarding HRCT findings in LCH?

A Early stage involvement shows honeycombing.

B In children under the age of 10 it may spontaneously regress.

C Pulmonary involvement is unusual.

D Pulmonary involvement represents a poor prognosis.

E The costophrenic angles are commonly involved.

Answer on page 336

MODULE 5

Paediatrics

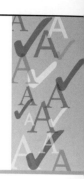

ANSWERS

QUESTION 1

ANSWER: D

Subdural haemorrhage is the most common finding and, in the absence of a clear mechanism of injury, is highly suspicious for NAI.

Reference: *Grainger & Allison's* 5e, pp 1631–1632.

QUESTION 2

ANSWER: A

Only 5% of cases of gastroschisis are associated with other congenital anomalies.

Reference: *Grainger & Allison's* 5e, p 1488.

QUESTION 3

ANSWER: D

The neonatal chest radiograph differs from the infant; the ribs tend to be more horizontal, resulting in a cylindrical shape and the CTR can be as large as 65%.

Reference: *Grainger & Allison's* 5e, pp 1461–1462.

QUESTION 4

ANSWER: E

If a line does not intersect the capitellum on all views a dislocation should be suspected.

Reference: *Grainger & Allison's* 5e, pp 1613–1614.

QUESTION 5

ANSWER: E

Imaging is best performed in the prone position with a horizontal beam. Infants with an H-type fistula will have gas-filled bowel loops.

Reference: *Grainger & Allison's* 5e, pp 1488–1489.

QUESTION 6

ANSWER: B

The sagittal suture is the most commonly affected in primary craniosynostosis. Involvement of the coronal suture (in brachycephaly) is often associated with clinical syndromes.

Reference: *Grainger & Allison's* 5e, pp 1674–1676.

QUESTION 7

ANSWER: C

A micturating cystogram is indicated if the infant is under the age of 6 months, but is not a requirement if the infant is > 6 months unless there is an abnormal US or DMSA.

Reference: *Grainger & Allison's* 5e, pp 1537–1539. *Guidelines for UTI's in children* - NICE 2007.

QUESTION 8

ANSWER: D

Sickle cell anaemia needs to be excluded from this child's history. Up to 70% of osteomyelitis seen in sickle cell anaemia is due to *Salmonella*.

Reference: *Grainger & Allison's* 5e, p 1603.

QUESTION 9

ANSWER: B

The radiographic features of TTN include hyperaeration of the lungs with an increase in pulmonary interstitial markings. Resolution should be seen clinically and radiographically within 48–72 hours.

Reference: *Grainger & Allison's* 5e, pp 1463–1464.

QUESTION 10

ANSWER: C

Calcification is common and present in 50% of plain abdominal radiographs. Hepatoblastoma tends not to be multifocal; this would make hepatocellular carcinoma a more likely diagnosis.

Reference: *Grainger & Allison's* 5e, p 1520.

QUESTION 11

ANSWER: E

Ultrasound criteria include canal length > 16 mm, transverse pyloric diameter > 11 mm, muscle wall thickening > 2.5 mm and increased gastric motility. A pylorus that does not open is associated with hypertrophic stenosis; however, it may also be seen in pylorospasm.

Reference: *Grainger & Allison's* 5e, p 1505.

QUESTION 12

ANSWER: C

If a paediatric posterior mediastinal mass contains calcification, it is most likely to be a sympathetic chain tumour.

Reference: *Grainger & Allison's* 5e, pp 1479–1480.

QUESTION 13

ANSWER: D

The history suggests posterior urethral valves. The most appropriate first line imaging is a micturating cystourethrogram with oblique views.

Reference: *Grainger & Allison's* 5e, p1546–1547

QUESTION 14

ANSWER: E

Wilms' tumours are associated with nephroblastomatosis; however, nephroblastomatosis is nonenhancing.

Reference: *Grainger & Allison's* 5e, pp 1559–1561.

QUESTION 15

ANSWER: E

VSD is the only option that presents as acyanotic heart disease with pulmonary plethora.

Reference: *Grainger & Allison's* 5e, pp 452–453.

QUESTION 16

ANSWER: C

HRCT should ideally be performed in order to determine the extent and distribution of disease. Breathing can be controlled under anaesthesia to ensure adequate inspiration.

Reference: *Grainger & Allison's* 5e, p 1483.

QUESTION 17

ANSWER: C

Children may also get spinal cord injury without radiographic abnormality (SCIWORA) as the ligaments are lax; therefore, MRI may be necessary.

Reference: *Grainger & Allison's* 5e, pp 1696–1697.

QUESTION 18

ANSWER: B

Other features include a 'bone within bone' appearance, 'hair on end' appearance with widening of diplopic spaces in the skull and generalised osteopenia.

Reference: Tyler PA, Madani G, Chaudhuri R, et al. The radiological appearances of thalassaemia. *Clin Radiol* 2006;61(1):40–52.

QUESTION 19

ANSWER: D

The typical imaging algorithm for children suspected of a primary bone malignancy includes plain radiograph, MRI to cover the entire bone involved by the lesion, bone scintigraphy to look for skeletal metastases and a CT chest for pulmonary metastases.

Reference: *Grainger & Allison's* 5e, p 1646.

QUESTION 20

ANSWER: A

Malrotation predisposes patients to midgut volvulus, giving rise to the 'corkscrew' pattern.

Reference: *Grainger & Allison's* 5e, p 1491.

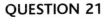

QUESTION 21

ANSWER: B

A contrast enema will demonstrate a microcolon, with reflux into the terminal ileum which should be small in calibre and demonstrate pellets of meconium. Reflux into the more proximal ileum will demonstrate a dilated ileum.

Reference: *Grainger & Allison's* 5e, p 1497.

QUESTION 22

ANSWER: C

It is common to see calcification within the inflammatory mass as well as associated ureteric calcification. The abscess cavities are low attenuation on CT, with surrounding rim enhancement.

Reference: *Grainger & Allison's* 5e, p 1552.

QUESTION 23

ANSWER: A

ADEM can occur following a viral illness and is classically a monophasic illness that occurs in multiple sites within the brain and the spinal cord. Multiple sclerosis is a possible diagnosis; however, the clinical history makes this far less likely.

Reference: *Grainger & Allison's* 5e, pp 1695–1696.

QUESTION 24

ANSWER: A

Pleural effusions are unusual in the newborn; other causes include hydrops fetalis, cardiac failure and perinatal infection.

Reference: *Grainger & Allison's* 5e, p 1467.

QUESTION 25

ANSWER: E

If an infant suffers hypoxic damage at term, the areas most affected are those that are most metabolically active. These include the putamen, thalami and adjacent white matter.

Reference: *Grainger & Allison's* 5e, p 1689.

QUESTION 26

ANSWER: D

The typical ultrasound findings represent bile duct lakes with the portal vein seen as a central echogenic dot.

Reference: *Grainger & Allison's* 5e, pp 1516–1518.

QUESTION 27

ANSWER: A

The age of the child and the description of the tumour fit best with a choroid plexus tumour. Another diagnosis that should be considered is medulloblastoma, but this tends to occur in an older age group with peak presentation at 7 years.

Reference: *Grainger & Allison's* 5e, p 1678.

QUESTION 28

ANSWER: D

The differential diagnoses for a lesion within the posterior elements of a vertebral body include osteoid osteoma, osteoblastoma and an aneurysmal bone cyst.

Reference: *Grainger & Allison's* 5e, pp 1640–1642.

QUESTION 29

ANSWER: C

Congenital hernias are usually Bochdalek hernias. Morgagni hernias are usually right-sided, anterior and smaller and tend to occur later on in life.

Reference: *Grainger & Allison's* 5e, p 1467.

QUESTION 30

ANSWER: D

An echocardiogram can be used but it becomes more difficult to assess the coarctation repair as the child gets older.

Reference: *Grainger & Allison's* 5e, p 457.

QUESTION 31

ANSWER: A

Over half of abdominal masses originate from the genitourinary tract. Hydronephrosis makes up 25% of these. A multicystic dysplastic kidney makes up about 15%; the remaining diagnoses rarely present as cystic masses.

Reference: Chapman S, Nakielny R. *Aids to Radiological Differential Diagnosis*, 5th edition (Edinburgh: Saunders, 2003), pp 361–362, 370.

QUESTION 32

ANSWER: A

Subchondral lucency is the earliest feature of Perthes' disease and is known as the 'crescent sign'. Fragmentation and sclerosis of the femoral head are chronic features of Perthes'.

Reference: *Grainger & Allison's* 5e, p 1592.

QUESTION 33

ANSWER: D

Medulloblastoma is the most common posterior fossa tumour in children, accounting for 30–40%.

Reference: *Grainger & Allison's* 5e, p 1677.

QUESTION 34

ANSWER: D

The alpha angle should measure > 60°. An alpha angle of 55°–59° at 4 weeks can be physiologically normal; however, follow-up is advised.

Reference: *Grainger & Allison's* 5e, pp 1588–1591.

QUESTION 35

ANSWER: B

Distal intestinal obstruction presents in 10-15% of older CF sufferers and can be potentially fatal. Treatment is with oral Gastrografin and a Gastrografin enema.

Reference: *Grainger & Allison's* 5e, p 1509.

QUESTION 36

ANSWER: D

LCH may be focal or systemic but commonly affects skin, bone and lung.

References: *Grainger & Allison's* 5e, p 1782.
Kilborn TN, Teh J, Goodman TR. Paediatric manifestations of Langerhans cell histiocytosis: a review of the clinical and radiological manifestations. *Clin Radiol* 2003;58:269–278.

QUESTION 37

ANSWER: C

The fact that the condition is unilateral and detected during the antenatal scan makes C the most likely diagnosis. The remaining diagnoses are most often bilateral or diagnosed later in life.

Reference: *Grainger & Allison's* 5e, p 1555.

QUESTION 38

ANSWER: B

The Dandy Walker malformation is a cystic dilatation of the fourth ventricle. The main differential is a posterior fossa arachnoid cyst; however, this does not communicate with the fourth ventricle.

Reference: *Grainger & Allison's* 5e, pp 1655–1656, 1657–8.

QUESTION 39

ANSWER: B

Indications for a DTPA scan also include follow-up of renal transplant, renography with captopril stimulation and postoperative evaluation of a collecting system.

Reference: *Grainger & Allison's* 5e, p 1538.

QUESTION 40

ANSWER: A

Osteochondritis dissecans is a subchondral defect which may lead to separation of the subchondral bone.

Reference: *Grainger & Allison's* 5e, p 1617.

QUESTION 41

ANSWER: A

The capitellum starts to ossify around 3 months, the radial head and medial epicondyle around 5 years, the trochlea around 8 years and the lateral condyle and the olecranon around 10 years.

Reference: *Grainger & Allison's* 5e, p 1613.

QUESTION 42

ANSWER: D

Ultrasound is a first line imaging investigation, and is very useful in picking up early stage liver cirrhosis and gallstones.

Reference: *Grainger & Allison's* 5e, pp 1510–1511.

QUESTION 43

ANSWER: E

The umbilical arterial line should lie between T6 and T10 or between L3 and L5, in order to avoid the origins of the spinal and renal arteries.

Reference: *Grainger & Allison's* 5e, pp 1462–1463.

QUESTION 44

ANSWER: A

Normal suture widths are greater than 10 mm at birth, 3 mm at 2 years, and 2 mm at 3 years.

Reference: Chapman & Nakielny, *Aids to Radiological Differential Diagnosis*, p 382.

QUESTION 45

ANSWER: B

The classic triad of 'shaken baby syndrome' is retinal haemorrhages, subdural haemorrhage and encephalopathy.

Reference: *Grainger & Allison's* 5e, p 1697.

QUESTION 46

ANSWER: E

RPD is diagnosed when there is calyceal dilatation with a renal pelvis that measures greater than 5 mm in the second trimester or 10 mm in the third trimester. No ureteric dilatation should be seen.

Reference: *Grainger & Allison's* 5e, p 1541.

QUESTION 47

ANSWER: B

The duodenum and jejunum are the commonest sites of involvement. However, intussusceptions tend to be located in the ileoileal region and are usually transient.

Reference: *Grainger & Allison's* 5e, p 1502.

QUESTION 48

ANSWER: B

Eighty per cent of infants with persistent neonatal jaundice will have biliary atresia or neonatal hepatitis. Decompression of biliary atresia is important for preventing cirrhosis.

Reference: *Grainger & Allison's* 5e, p1514–1515

QUESTION 49

ANSWER: B

Horseshoe kidney is the most common fusion abnormality and arises when both lower poles have fused together. Crossed fused ectopia occurs when one kidney is displaced across the midline and fused inferiorly to the other kidney, but both ureters enter the bladder in a normal position.

Reference: *Grainger & Allison's* 5e, p 1534.

QUESTION 50

ANSWER: D

Increased signal within the subdural space relative to CSF on both T1w and T2w images is consistent with a subdural empyema. This is likely to require urgent drainage, whereas subdural effusions do not need surgical treatment and will resolve as the meningitis is treated.

Reference: *Grainger & Allison's* 5e, pp 1692–1693.

QUESTION 51

ANSWER: A

The pelvic radiographs are taken in an AP projection.

Reference: *Grainger & Allison's* 5e, p 1593.

QUESTION 52

ANSWER: D

Meconium aspiration syndrome has a mortality of 25%. Pneumothorax and pneumomediastinum are commonly seen.

Reference: *Grainger & Allison's* 5e, p 1466.

QUESTION 53

ANSWER: A

The boot shaped heart is seen secondary to the right ventricular hypertrophy.

Reference: *Grainger & Allison's* 5e, p 460.

QUESTION 54

ANSWER: B

Ebstein's anomaly is a congenital abnormality of the tricuspid valve. It results in tricuspid regurgitation and atrialisation of the right ventricle. It is usually associated with an atrial septal defect (ASD), and a right-to-left shunt with cyanosis.

Reference: *Grainger & Allison's* 5e, p 464.

QUESTION 55

ANSWER: C

The upper ureter usually enters as an ureterocele, but the lower pole ureter is the one more frequently affected by reflux. Reflux is rarely seen to the upper moiety.

Reference: *Grainger & Allison's* 5e, pp 1548–1549.

QUESTION 56

ANSWER: D

The findings are all consistent with renal vein thrombosis, which can be seen in the dehydrated septic neonate. Ultrasound changes of acute tubular necrosis are usually symmetrical.

Reference: *Grainger & Allison's* 5e, p 1542.

QUESTION 57

ANSWER: A

JIA is a cause of a widened intercondylar notch secondary to joint effusions and synovial hypertrophy.

Reference: *Grainger & Allison's* 5e, pp 1595–1597.

QUESTION 58

ANSWER: A

Portal venous gas is seen in 10% of cases and is not always fatal. Its disappearance may indicate impending perforation.

Reference: *Grainger & Allison's* 5e, pp 1493–1494.

QUESTION 59

ANSWER: D

The success rate is 60% with a perforation rate of 5%.

Reference: *Grainger & Allison's* 5e, p 1497.

QUESTION 60

ANSWER: E

Eisenmenger's syndrome occurs in adulthood. The duct and the pulmonary arteries may become calcified.

Reference: *Grainger & Allison's* 5e, pp 452, 459.

QUESTION 61

ANSWER: A

Standard radiographs for craniosynostosis assessment includes Townes', AP and lateral projections.

Reference: *Grainger & Allison's* 5e, pp 1674–1675.

QUESTION 62

ANSWER: C

The commonest cause of vertebral body collapse in children is Langerhans cell histiocytosis, giving the characteristic 'vertebra plana' appearance.

Reference: Kilborn TN, Teh J, Goodman TR. Paediatric manifestations of Langerhans cell histiocytosis: a review of the clinical and radiological findings. *Clin Radiol* 2003;58(4): 269–278.

QUESTION 63

ANSWER: C

The liver in the newborn is less reflective than the kidney up to the age of 3–4 months. A patent umbilical vein after 2–3 weeks is not usual and is associated with portal hypertension.

Reference: *Grainger & Allison's* 5e, pp 1513–1514.

QUESTION 64

ANSWER: C

Calcification on CT is seen in up to 85% of children with neuroblastoma and bone metastases are also more common with this tumour. It is usual for both tumours to enhance less than the surrounding renal parenchyma and neuroblastomas tend to encase vessels, rather than displace them.

Reference: *Grainger & Allison's* 5e, pp 1563, 1647.

QUESTION 65

ANSWER: D

In children the majority of Meckel's diverticula contain intestinal mucosa.

Reference: *Grainger & Allison's* 5e, p 674. Chapman S, Nakielny R, p 271.

QUESTION 66

ANSWER: D

Skip lesions and short segment disease are unusual and a biopsy is required for definitive diagnosis. The catheter balloon should never be inflated, as this runs the risk of perforation.

Reference: *Grainger & Allison's* 5e, p 1495.

QUESTION 67

ANSWER: C

Fractures to the outer third of the clavicle metaphysis, ribs, scapula, sternal and spinous process all have a high specificity for NAI.

Reference: *Grainger & Allison's* 5e, pp 1623–1628.

QUESTION 68

ANSWER: C

Both testicular and Wilms' tumours metastasise to lungs; however, the age of the patient is highly atypical for a testicular tumour (more common in adolescence and young adulthood).

Reference: *Grainger & Allison's* 5e, p 1481.

QUESTION 69

ANSWER: A

Round pneumonia tends to have ill-defined margins, lacks an air bronchogram and resolves quickly with treatment. Correlative history is crucial.

Reference: *Grainger & Allison's* 5e, p 1471.

QUESTION 70

ANSWER: A

Subependymal nodules are the most common neurological abnormality, seen in 85–95% of patients.

Reference: *Grainger & Allison's* 5e, pp 1665–1666.

QUESTION 71

ANSWER: C

Typical radiographic features include posterior vertebral body scalloping, bullet-shaped vertebrae and a decreased interpedicular distance.

Reference: *Grainger & Allison's* 5e, p 1572.

QUESTION 72

ANSWER: B

Trisomy 21 is seen in approximately 30% of patients with duodenal atresia/stenosis and an annular pancreas.

Reference: *Grainger & Allison's* 5e, p 1492.

QUESTION 73

ANSWER: C

Studies have demonstrated that effective reduction and a lower radiation dose are achieved by using air reduction rather than barium.

References: *Grainger & Allison's* 5e, pp 1499–1501.
Heenan SD, Kyriou J, Fitzgerald M, et al. Effective dose at pneumatic reduction of paediatric intussusception. *Clin Radiol* 2000;55(11):811–816.

QUESTION 74

ANSWER: D

Reference: *Grainger & Allison's* 5e, pp 1599–1600.

QUESTION 75

ANSWER: B

A nasogastric tube is a very useful tool in suspected OA, but if the tube passes into the stomach it may have entered through a fistulous connection. However, if an NG tube curls up in a proximal air-filled oesophagus, OA is highly likely.

Reference: *Grainger & Allison's* 5e, pp 1488–1489.

QUESTION 76

ANSWER: E

Hilar enlargement results from enlarged pulmonary vasculature and is a sign of pulmonary hypertension.

Reference: *Grainger & Allison's* 5e, p 1482.

QUESTION 77

ANSWER: D

CCAM may present in a similar manner, but as the mass becomes aerated it appears as a multicystic, fluid-filled mass.

Reference: *Grainger & Allison's* 5e, p 1468.

QUESTION 78

ANSWER: B

Optic pathway gliomas are the most commonly seen intracranial abnormality in NF1. The commonest location in children is within the optic nerve rather than the chiasm.

Reference: *Grainger & Allison's* 5e, pp 1663–1664.

QUESTION 79

ANSWER: C

During the first 6 months of life, brain maturation is easiest to follow on T1w images, where the appearance of myelin is bright. By 10 months the T1w images will have an almost adult appearance, and further changes are easier to assess using the T2w images.

Reference: *Grainger & Allison's* 5e, pp 1653–1655.

QUESTION 80

ANSWER: B

Pulmonary involvement is seen in 42% of patients but it doesn't necessarily represent a poor prognosis. Reticular or reticulonodular shadowing is seen predominantly within the upper and mid zones, typically with sparing of the costophrenic angles.

Reference: Kilborn TN, Teh J, Goodman TR. Paediatric manifestations of Langerhans cell histiocytosis: a review of the clinical and radiological findings. *Clin Radiol* 2003;58 (4):269–278.

Central Nervous and Head & Neck

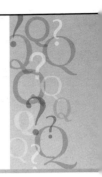

QUESTIONS

QUESTION 1

A 42-year-old woman with known Wegener's granulomatosis presents with pain on moving her left eye. On examination she has left-sided proptosis and pain on all eye movements. CT of the orbits demonstrates inflammation of the left-sided extraocular muscles and their tendinous insertions with enhancement postcontrast. There is also increased attenuation within the retrobulbar fat as well as enlargement of the lacrimal gland. What is the most likely diagnosis?

  A Capillary haemangioma
  B Graves' disease
  C Orbital lymphoma
  D Orbital pseudotumour
  E Retinoblastoma

Answer on page 378

QUESTION 2

A 33-year-old HIV-positive woman presents with increasing headache and confusion. On examination she is pyrexial and has left leg and right facial weakness. A CT head demonstrates multiple lesions measuring between 2 and 4 cm which are predominantly situated at the corticomedullary junction. These lesions have a thin enhancing rim as well as associated oedema and local mass effect. Which one of the following is the most likely diagnosis?

A Cryptococcosis

B Histiocytosis

C HIV encephalopathy

D Multiple cerebral metastases

E Toxoplasmosis

Answer on page 378

QUESTION 3

A 28-year-old woman suffers a 1-week episode of diarrhoea and vomiting due to the Norwalk virus. She is noted by her boyfriend to be increasingly lethargic at home and is unable to tolerate oral fluids. She then becomes confused and agitated and suffers a generalised tonic clonic seizure. Which one of the following radiological findings is most likely?

A Focal high signal on FLAIR images within the right cerebellar hemisphere

B Focal ovoid lesions of high FLAIR signal in the periventricular white matter

C High signal on FLAIR images in the occipital lobes

D High signal on FLAIR images in the parasagittal cortex bilaterally

E Loss of grey–white matter differentiation in the region of the basal ganglia and insula bilaterally

Answer on page 378

QUESTION 4

A 41-year-old woman presents with a 2-day history of disorientation and headache. She describes general malaise over the preceding week. No localising neurological signs are elicited on examination. She has a CT head which is normal, but her symptoms deteriorate and she has a generalised tonic clonic seizure the following day. Which of the following findings would you expect to see on a repeat CT scan?

A A thin fluid collection in the interhemispheric fissure which has an enhancing rim

B Bilateral rims of low attenuation overlying the temporoparietal cortex

C Low attenuation in the frontal and temporal lobes with patchy gyriform enhancement postcontrast

D Multiple large low attenuation areas within the white matter

E Ovoid lesions of high T2 signal in the periventricular white matter orientated perpendicular to the lateral ventricles

Answer on page 379

QUESTION 5

A 12-year-old child is suspected to have a diagnosis of neurofibromatosis. Which one of the following radiological findings would favour a diagnosis of neurofibromatosis type 1 over neurofibromatosis type 2?

A Bilateral acoustic neuromas

B Leptomeningeal angiomas

C Multiple meningiomas

D Sphenoid wing hypoplasia

E Spinal ependymoma

Answer on page 379

QUESTION 6

A 30-year-old man has a CT head to investigate headaches. This shows a low attenuation mass in the left temporoparietal region which has similar density to CSF and shows no enhancement following contrast administration. Which one of the following radiological findings would support a diagnosis of epidermoid cyst rather than arachnoid cyst?

A High signal on diffusion-weighted MRI
B High signal on FLAIR MRI
C Low signal on diffusion-weighted MRI
D Thinning of the overlying bone
E Well-defined margins

Answer on page 379

QUESTION 7

A 44-year-old woman has a history of pain and swelling in her left cheek, particularly after eating. Her GP is suspicious that she has a parotid duct calculus and refers her for sialography. Which one of the following statements is true regarding sialography?

A Approximately 10 mL contrast is usually required to fill the parotid duct and branches.
B High-osmolar contrast media are contraindicated.
C It is contraindicated in acute infection.
D Pain post-procedure warrants further investigation.
E The orifice of the parotid duct is adjacent to the second upper premolar.

Answer on page 379

QUESTION 8

A young patient undergoes CT of the paranasal sinuses. The main finding is an enhancing nasal mass with widening of the left pterygopalatine fissure. What is the most likely diagnosis?

A Adenoid cystic carcinoma

B Angiofibroma

C Angiosarcoma

D Inverting papilloma

E Lymphoma

Answer on page 380

QUESTION 9

A 76-year-old man presents to the Emergency Department with headache and vomiting. He gives a 2-month history of transient episodes of limb weakness. His blood pressure is normal. A CT head is performed and shows several areas of frontal and parietal subcortical high attenuation. The ventricles and extra-axial CSF spaces appear normal. Which one of the following is the most likely diagnosis?

A Amyloid angiopathy

B Haemorrhagic infarcts

C Hypertensive haemorrhages

D Multifocal lymphoma

E Subarachnoid haemorrhages

Answer on page 380

QUESTION 10

A 22-month-old child with developmental delay presents with seizures. The MRI findings include hydrocephalus with a markedly dilated fourth ventricle and hypoplasia of the cerebellar vermis. Which one of the following is the most likely diagnosis?

A Chiari II malformation

B Dandy-Walker malformation

C Encephalocele

D Holoprosencephaly

E Joubert's syndrome

Answer on page 380

QUESTION 11

A 5-year-old boy presents with rapidly progressive right-sided proptosis. On examination, he is noted to have lateral deviation of the right eye but visual acuity is normal. CT of the orbits reveals a large, isodense mass in the superomedial right orbit. The extraocular muscles cannot be seen separately and there is destruction of the medial wall of the bony orbit. The mass displays uniform enhancement postcontrast. What is the most likely diagnosis?

A Capillary haemangioma

B Dermoid cyst

C Intraconal schwannoma

D Retinoblastoma

E Rhabdomyosarcoma

Answer on page 380

QUESTION 12

A 46-year-old woman presents with a painful left eye. She has enophthalmos on clinical examination. CT reveals a mass arising from the greater wing of the left sphenoid with some underlying bone destruction. The mass is poorly marginated and infiltrating the intraconal compartment. What is the most likely diagnosis?

A Caroticocavernous fistula

B Lymphoma

C Metastatic breast carcinoma

D Orbital dermoid

E Orbital varix

Answer on page 380

QUESTION 13

A 46-year-old woman presents with an insidious onset of weakness and numbness in her lower limbs, associated with worsening mid thoracic back pain. MRI of the spine reveals a well-defined intradural, extramedullary mass in the mid-thoracic region. The mass is isointense to the spinal cord on both T1w and T2w images and there is uniform enhancement postcontrast. What is the most likely diagnosis?

A Chordoma

B Dermoid cyst

C Meningioma

D Metastasis

E Multiple myeloma

Answer on page 381

QUESTION 14

A 9-year-old girl is referred for a neck ultrasound to investigate a superficial swelling at the angle of her left mandible. The scan reveals a well-defined, anechoic lesion anterior to the left sternocleidomastoid muscle with posterior acoustic enhancement. What is the most likely diagnosis?

A Pseudoaneurysm of the left common carotid artery

B Ranula

C Second branchial cleft cyst

D Third branchial cleft cyst

E Thyroglossal duct cyst

Answer on page 381

QUESTION 15

A 33-year-old woman presents to the Emergency Department with a reduced conscious level. She has been generally unwell with fever, malaise and a dry cough for several weeks and more recently has developed a left facial nerve palsy. An MRI brain reveals nodular thickening and enhancement of the dura and leptomeninges. There is also enhancement of the optic tracts and optic chiasm, as well as the pituitary infundibulum. A few small foci of high T2 signal are demonstrated in the periventricular white matter. What is the most likely diagnosis?

A Multiple sclerosis

B Langerhans cell histiocytosis

C Progressive multifocal leucoencephalopathy

D Sarcoidosis

E Wilson's disease

Answer on page 381

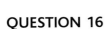

QUESTION 16

A 21-year-old man has facial and mandibular radiographs following minor trauma. These show no evidence of fracture, however there are multiple dense bony lesions arising from the paranasal sinuses and the angle and ramus of the mandible. These lesions are entirely asymptomatic. Which one of the following conditions may be associated with these findings?

A Gardner's syndrome

B Gorlin-Goltz syndrome

C Juvenile polyposis

D Klippel-Feil syndrome

E Turner's syndrome

Answer on page 381

QUESTION 17

A 77-year-old gentleman suffers a ruptured abdominal aortic aneurysm for which he undergoes emergency surgery. Early in the postoperative period he develops acute lower back pain and is incontinent. An urgent MRI is performed. What are the most likely radiological findings?

A Enhancing, heterogeneous intramedullary mass lesion

B Extradural collection with peripheral enhancement

C Focal high T2 signal within the spinal cord with mild cord swelling

D Large central disc herniation at the affected level with associated high T2 signal within the cord

E Marked diffuse swelling of the spinal cord at the affected level

Answer on page 382

QUESTION 18

A 68-year-old man presents with left facial weakness and a craggy parotid mass. Investigations reveal a left parotid tumour which is found to be an adenoid cystic carcinoma following surgical resection. Which one of the following statements is true regarding adenoid cystic carcinoma affecting the salivary glands?

A It has a propensity for perineural spread.

B It is a rapidly growing tumour.

C It is also known as Warthin's tumour.

D It is commonest in the parotid gland.

E It usually has the appearance of a multiloculated cyst on ultrasound.

Answer on page 382

QUESTION 19

A 40-year-old motorcyclist is brought to the Emergency Department following a road traffic accident. His GCS at the scene was 9 but has now dropped to 6. His CT head reveals multiple small hyperdense lesions at the corticomedullary junction and in both basal ganglia. His condition does not improve and his GCS drops further to 4. He remains in hospital and an MRI scan a month after his admission shows low signal foci on T2w images at the corticomedullary junction and in the basal ganglia. What is the most likely diagnosis?

A Diffuse axonal injury

B Extensive subarachnoid haemorrhage

C Hypoxic cerebral injury

D Multiple haemorrhagic contusions

E Venous infarction

Answer on page 382

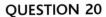

QUESTION 20

A 33-year-old man undergoes an MRI brain to investigate worsening headaches, which he gets predominantly in the mornings. Findings include a lobulated mass in the fourth ventricle, which extends via the foramen of Magendie into the cisterna magna. The mass is predominantly low signal on T1w images and high on T2w images. Mild heterogeneous enhancement is seen postcontrast. What is the most likely diagnosis?

A Choroid plexus carcinoma

B Choroid plexus papilloma

C Ependymoma

D Meningioma

E Myxopapillary ependymoma

Answer on page 382

QUESTION 21

A 76-year-old man who has been previously well attends for a CT head as part of investigations for dementia. This reveals severe atrophy of the anterior temporal lobes, more marked on the right side. Which one of the following conditions is this most suggestive of?

A Alzheimer's disease

B Encephalitis

C Lewy body dementia

D Multisystem atrophy

E Pick's disease

Answer on page 383

QUESTION 22

A 53-year-old man is admitted with fever, headache and drowsiness. A CT head reveals a low attenuation lesion at the corticomedullary junction of the left frontal lobe with an enhancing rim and some surrounding low attenuation change. Opacification of his paranasal sinuses is also noted. What is the most likely diagnosis?

A Metastasis

B Primary cerebral lymphoma

C Pyogenic abscess

D Toxoplasmosis

E Tuberculous abscess

Answer on page 383

QUESTION 23

A GP requests your advice regarding an 18-month-old girl whose mother has noticed that her left pupil appears white. The GP has performed ophthalmoscopy and is suspicious that there is a retinal mass. Which one of the following is the investigation of choice?

A CT orbits

B MRI orbits

C Orbital radiographs

D Repeat ophthalmoscopy by ophthalmologist

E Ultrasound

Answer on page 383

QUESTION 24

An 82-year-old woman who was previously well has had several falls in the past 2–3 months. She has become increasingly confused but there are no localising neurological signs on physical examination. Which one of the following is the most likely finding on CT?

A High attenuation in both Sylvian fissures, the basal cisterns and the lateral ventricles.

B High attenuation overlying the right frontoparietal cortex and extending into the interhemispheric space with midline shift to the left.

C Mixed attenuation areas overlying both hemispheres with normal ventricles and no midline shift.

D High attenuation lentiform collection overlying the left temporal region with effacement of the left lateral ventricle.

E Superficial areas of low density in the right frontotemporal region, containing small foci of high attenuation.

Answer on page 383

QUESTION 25

A 7-year-old boy is referred from the paediatric clinic for an MRI brain to investigate learning difficulties and abnormal gait. The MRI reveals high T2 signal in the splenium and posterior body of the corpus callosum as well as in the peritrigonal white matter. There is marginal enhancement at the anterior edge of the abnormal area. Which one of the following is the most likely diagnosis?

A Adrenoleukodystrophy

B Alexander disease

C Kearns-Sayer syndrome

D Krabbe's leukodystrophy

E Maple syrup urine disease

Answer on page 384

QUESTION 26

A 52-year-old woman is referred for a neck ultrasound by her GP. She was found to be hypercalcaemic on recent routine blood tests. Which one of the following findings would support the presence of a parathyroid adenoma?

A A well-defined hyperechoic mass posterior to the thyroid gland
B A well-defined hypoechoic mass posterior to the thyroid gland
C A well-defined hyperechoic mass anterior to the thyroid gland
D An ill-defined hyperechoic mass anterior to the thyroid gland
E An ill-defined hypoechoic mass posterior to the thyroid gland

Answer on page 384

QUESTION 27

A 3-year-old boy has an MRI brain which shows descent of the cerebellar tonsils below the foramen magnum. Which one of the following is more likely to suggest a Chiari I rather than a Chiari II malformation?

A Craniosynostosis
B Elongation of the medulla
C Hydrocephalus
D Myelomeningocoele
E Tectal beaking

Answer on page 384

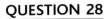

QUESTION 28

A 19-year-old HIV-positive man is admitted with headaches, confusion and disorientation. He is mildly pyrexial. A CT brain reveals multiple hypodensities, particularly in the brainstem and in the periventricular white matter. There is some ependymal enhancement postcontrast. What is the most likely cause for these findings?

A CMV encephalitis

B Cryptococcosis

C HIV encephalitis

D Toxoplasmosis

E Tuberculosis

Answer on page 385

QUESTION 29

A 35-year-old man is admitted from outpatient clinic with a history of worsening lower back pain and leg weakness. Plain lumbar radiographs reveal expansion of the spinal canal at L3–4 level. He has an urgent MRI which shows a lobulated extramedullary mass at this level, causing nerve root compression. The mass is hyperintense to the spinal cord on T2w images and there is an associated paravertebral mass. What is the most likely diagnosis?

A Astrocytoma

B Disc extrusion

C Ependymoma

D Meningioma

E Neurinoma

Answer on page 385

QUESTION 30

An 18-year-old man presents with increasing headaches. He has a CT brain which shows a solid hyperdense mass in the posterior aspect of the third ventricle, displaying avid enhancement postcontrast and associated with obstructive hydrocephalus. On MRI, the mass is hypointense on T2w images compared with grey matter and contains small cystic areas. There is also a smaller lesion with similar signal characteristics in the suprasellar region. The solid components of both lesions appear homogeneous and enhance avidly postcontrast. What is the most likely diagnosis?

A Colloid cyst

B Germinoma

C Pineoblastoma

D Pineocytoma

E Teratoma

Answer on page 385

QUESTION 31

A 56-year-old man who is known to drink excessive amounts of alcohol is admitted to the Emergency Department with a GCS of 10. His routine blood tests reveal profound hyponatraemia. He is treated and his serum sodium level is normal 2 days later. However, his GCS has dropped to 6. What are the most likely findings on MRI?

A Foci of high T2 signal at the corticomedullary junction

B Foci of high T2 signal in both cerebellar hemispheres and occipital lobes

C Herniation of the cerebellar tonsils through the foramen magnum

D High T2 signal in the pons, basal ganglia and thalami

E Loss of grey–white matter differentiation

Answer on page 385

QUESTION 32

A 67-year-old woman with known osteoarthritis presents with lower back pain radiating down her left leg. She has an MRI of the lumbar spine which shows a lesion at the L4–5 facet joint with compression of the thecal sac at this level. The lesion is of intermediate signal on T2w images and is displacing the ligamentum flavum. What is the most likely diagnosis?

A Astrocytoma

B Disc protrusion

C Ependymoma

D Osteophyte

E Synovial cyst

Answer on page 386

QUESTION 33

A previously well 70-year-old man is admitted with an acute onset of left-sided weakness and dysphasia. CT shows low attenuation in the right temporoparietal region with loss of normal grey–white matter differentiation. He undergoes an MRI brain one week later. What are the most likely radiological findings?

A High FLAIR signal in the right temporoparietal region with no enhancement seen postcontrast

B High T2 signal in the right temporoparietal region with gyriform enhancement seen postcontrast

C High T2 signal in the right temporoparietal region with no enhancement seen postcontrast

D Intermediate T2 signal in the right temporoparietal region with no enhancement seen postcontrast

E Uniformly high signal on gradient echo images in the right temporoparietal region

Answer on page 386

QUESTION 34

A 50-year-old man has a CT head after sustaining a head injury during a mechanical fall. The only positive finding is a large low attenuation lesion in the left middle cranial fossa which is well defined and of the same attenuation as CSF. There is some thinning of the overlying temporal bone. Which one of the following is the most likely diagnosis?

A Arachnoid cyst
B Cerebral infarct
C Colloid cyst
D Dermoid cyst
E Epidermoid cyst

Answer on page 386

QUESTION 35

A 22-year-old woman presents with visual loss and headaches. On examination, she has bilateral visual field defects and decreased visual acuity. CT reveals foci of calcification at both optic nerve heads. What is the most likely diagnosis?

A Choroidal haemangioma
B Drusen
C Leukaemia
D Optic neuritis
E Sclerosing endophthalmitis

Answer on page 386

QUESTION 36

A 12-year-old girl presents with a 3-week history of lower back pain, malaise and a low grade fever. A lateral lumbar spine radiograph shows features suspicious of discitis. Which one of the following findings would support tuberculous rather than pyogenic infection?

A Bony bridging of affected vertebrae
B Destruction of the adjacent endplates
C Large paravertebral abscess
D Marked bony sclerosis
E Preserved vertebral body height

Answer on page 387

QUESTION 37

A 55-year-old woman presents with pulsatile tinnitus in her right ear. She also complains of dizziness and on examination she has hearing loss on the right side. MRI shows a mass in the right jugular fossa which is of high signal on T2w images and contains several low signal areas. There is marked enhancement postcontrast. What is the most likely diagnosis?

A Acoustic neuroma
B Glomus jugulare
C Glomus tympanicum
D Meningioma
E Metastasis

Answer on page 387

QUESTION 38

A 6-year-old girl with several pigmented patches on her skin presents with deteriorating vision. An MRI brain shows fusiform expansion of both optic nerves, with enlargement of the optic foramina. In addition there are multiple small lesions in the basal ganglia and pons which are hyperintense on T2w images. What is the most likely diagnosis?

A Neurofibromatosis type 1 with optic nerve gliomas and cerebral hamartomas

B Neurofibromatosis type 2 with optic nerve gliomas and cerebral hamartomas

C Neurofibromatosis type 2 with optic nerve meningiomas and multiple schwannomas

D Tuberous sclerosis with cortical tubers and retinal hamartomas

E Tuberous sclerosis with subependymal and retinal hamartomas

Answer on page 387

QUESTION 39

A 61-year-old woman presents with a gradual loss of visual acuity in the left eye. She has left-sided proptosis on examination. A CT head postcontrast reveals thickening of the optic nerve/sheath complex with a 'tram-track' appearance. There is some associated calcification. What is the most likely diagnosis?

A Cavernous haemangioma

B Lymphoma

C Optic nerve glioma

D Optic nerve haemangioblastoma

E Optic nerve meningioma

Answer on page 387

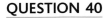

QUESTION 40

A 14-year-old girl with a kyphoscoliosis has multiple skin lesions which have been characterised as basal cell tumours. In addition she has had investigations which have revealed calcification of the falx and several bifid ribs. Which of the following findings would be most likely on a dental panoramic radiograph?

A A large well-defined lucency inferior to the inferior alveolar canal
B Multiple ill-defined lucent lesions
C Multiple sclerotic lesions, particularly around the angle of the mandible
D Multiple small periapical lucencies
E Multiple well-defined multiloculated lucencies

Answer on page 388

QUESTION 41

A 24-year-old man is referred to the neurology outpatient clinic with worsening headaches. Neurological examination reveals nystagmus and ataxia. A CT head shows a solitary, large, cystic mass in the posterior fossa with a solid, enhancing component. What is the most likely diagnosis?

A Colloid cyst
B Glioblastoma multiforme
C Haemangioblastoma
D Pilocytic astrocytoma
E Pleomorphic xanthoastrocytoma

Answer on page 388

QUESTION 42

A 32-year-old woman with a known history of excessive alcohol intake presents with a lump on the left side of her neck. She has an ultrasound scan which demonstrates a solitary nodule of mixed reflectivity in the left lobe of her thyroid which measures 3 cm in diameter. She also has several enlarged, uniformly hypoechoic cervical lymph nodes. On thyroid scintigraphy a low uptake region is seen corresponding to the site of the nodule. What is the most likely diagnosis?

A Colloid nodule

B De Quervain's thyroiditis

C Follicular carcinoma of thyroid

D Graves' disease

E Papillary carcinoma of thyroid

Answer on page 388

QUESTION 43

A 54-year-old man presents with headaches which are worse in the mornings. On examination, he has a bitemporal hemianopia. MRI reveals a predominantly solid suprasellar mass, which contains a small cystic component of high signal on T1w and T2w images. Intense enhancement of the solid component is seen following administration of intravenous gadolinium. Which one of the following is the most likely diagnosis?

A Craniopharyngioma

B Medulloblastoma

C Pituitary macroadenoma

D Pituitary microadenoma

E Rathke's cleft cyst

Answer on page 388

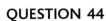

QUESTION 44

A 41-year-old woman has a 5-month history of left-sided tinnitus.
She undergoes an MRI scan which reveals a tumour arising from the left
cerebellopontine angle and extending into the internal auditory meatus. It has
mixed solid and cystic components. What is the most likely diagnosis?

A Epidermoid cyst

B Glomus tympanicum

C Haemangioma

D Meningioma

E Vestibular schwannoma

Answer on page 388

QUESTION 45

A 24-year-old woman presents to her GP with jaw stiffness and headaches.
Her partner complains that she grinds her teeth during the night. She attends
for an MRI scan to visualise the temporomandibular joints. Sequences are
performed with the mouth open and closed. Which of the following
radiological findings are most likely?

A Anterolateral displacement of the biconcave articular disc on mouth
closing

B Anteromedial displacement of the biconcave articular disc on mouth
opening

C Anteromedial displacement of the biconvex articular disc on mouth
opening

D Posterior displacement of the biconcave articular disc on mouth opening

E Posterior displacement of the biconvex articular disc on mouth opening

Answer on page 389

QUESTION 46

A 72-year-old man presented 4 days ago with right-sided weakness. CT at that time demonstrated an acute left frontoparietal haematoma. He now attends for an MRI brain. Which one of the following signal characteristics would you expect to see in the region of the haematoma?

A High signal on T1w and T2w images
B High signal on T1w and low signal on T2w images
C Low signal on T1w and T2w images
D Low signal on T1w and high signal on T2w images
E None of the above

Answer on page 389

QUESTION 47

A 9-month-old boy is noted to have an absent red reflex in his right eye, following a photograph taken by his family. An ophthalmologist confirms the presence of a retinal mass and a CT is requested. Which one of the following best describes the findings you would expect to see in a case of retinoblastoma on CT?

A Avidly enhancing, non-calcified retinal mass
B Avidly enhancing retinal mass with punctate calcification
C Hyperdense, non-calcified retinal mass
D Poorly enhancing, non-calcified retinal mass
E Poorly enhancing retinal mass with clumped calcification

Answer on page 389

QUESTION 48

An 82-year-old man presents to the Emergency Department with a 4-day history of right homonymous hemianopia and right arm weakness. A CT head demonstrates mild low density in the left parieto-occipital cortex and he is treated conservatively for a cerebral infarct. Which of the following would be consistent with a cerebral infarct on diffusion-weighted MR imaging (DWI) and apparent diffusion coefficient (ADC) map?

A High signal on ADC map and high signal on DWI after 1 week

B High signal on ADC map and low signal on DWI after 1 week

C Low signal on ADC map and high signal on DWI after 1 week

D Low signal on ADC map and high signal on DWI after 1 month

E Low signal on ADC map and low signal on DWI after 1 month

Answer on page 389

QUESTION 49

An 18-month-old child with a facial port wine stain presents with reduced movement on the left side and developmental delay. Her mother also reports left-sided focal seizures. What are the most likely radiological findings?

A Atrophy of the left cerebral hemisphere with enhancement overlying the left parietal cortex and enlargement of the right choroid plexus

B Atrophy of the right cerebral hemisphere with enhancement overlying the right parietal cortex and enlargement of the right choroid plexus

C Cystic dilatation of the fourth ventricle with hypoplasia of the vermis and hydrocephalus

D Hydrocephalus, inferior displacement of the cerebellar tonsils and elongation of the fourth ventricle

E Multiple small calcified subependymal nodules, a partly cystic mass at the foramen of Monro and several retinal lesions

Answer on page 389

QUESTION 50

A 44-year-old HIV-positive woman is admitted to hospital with worsening headaches and drowsiness. CT reveals several ovoid high attenuation lesions in the periventricular white matter and the basal ganglia. Some of the lesions appear to be abutting the ventricles. The lesions display homogeneous enhancement postcontrast although some of the larger ones have a low attenuation centre. There is no evidence of haemorrhage or calcification. Which one of the following is the most likely diagnosis?

A Multiple metastases
B Multiple pyogenic abscesses
C Multiple tuberculous abscesses
D Primary cerebral lymphoma
E Toxoplasmosis

Answer on page 390

QUESTION 51

A 63-year-old previously fit and well woman presents to her optician with loss of vision in her left eye. On examination, the visual acuity in the left eye is markedly reduced and the vitreous appears opaque. After ophthalmology review, an MRI is performed and reveals a soft tissue mass on the wall of the globe which is of high signal on T1w images and low signal on T2w images. What is the most likely diagnosis?

A Cavernous haemangioma
B Ocular metastasis
C Pseudotumour
D Retinoblastoma
E Uveal melanoma

Answer on page 390

QUESTION 52

A 37-year-old man is brought to the Emergency Department with extensive facial injuries following a bicycle accident. Facial radiographs demonstrate multiple fractures. Which one of the following descriptions of Le Fort fractures is correct?

A Le Fort I: bilateral fractures of the rami of the mandible

B Le Fort I: fractures of the nasal bridge and medial orbital walls

C Le Fort II: bilateral fractures of the rami of the mandible and both zygomatic arches

D Le Fort II: fractures through the nasal bridge, lacrimal bones and medial orbital walls extending to the pterygoid plates

E Le Fort III: fractures through the nasal bridge, lacrimal bones and medial orbital walls extending to the pterygoid plates

Answer on page 390

QUESTION 53

A 21-year-old man has an ultrasound of the abdomen which shows bilateral renal masses and several pancreatic cysts. A diagnosis of von Hippel Lindau disease is being considered. The presence of which of the following intracranial tumours would be strongly supportive of this diagnosis?

A Astrocytoma

B Craniopharyngioma

C Haemangioblastoma

D Medulloblastoma

E Optic nerve glioma

Answer on page 390

QUESTION 54

A 65-year-old woman sees her GP with diarrhoea, palpitations and fatigue. Clinical examination of her neck is normal, but her thyroid function tests are consistent with hyperthyroidism and she is referred for thyroid scintigraphy. Which one of the following statements is true regarding radionuclide thyroid imaging?

A Iodine 123 is taken up by the salivary glands.

B If iodine 123 is used, imaging should be performed immediately after the injection.

C If Tc-99m pertechnetate is used, imaging should be performed 4–6 hours after the injection.

D Increased uptake may be seen in the pyramidal lobe in normal individuals.

E It is contraindicated in patients with known parathyroid malignancy.

Answer on page 390

QUESTION 55

A 32-year-old woman presents with infertility and irregular periods. Investigations performed by her GP demonstrate a markedly elevated prolactin level. What would be the most likely MRI finding?

A A 6-mm avidly enhancing mass in the posterior pituitary

B A 6-mm poorly enhancing mass in the anterior pituitary

C A 6-mm poorly enhancing mass in the posterior pituitary

D A 20-mm avidly enhancing mass in the anterior pituitary

E A 20-mm avidly enhancing mass in the posterior pituitary

Answer on page 391

QUESTION 56

A 65-year-old man undergoes a CT head as part of a dementia screen. This shows a well-defined high attenuation mass peripherally in the right parietal lobe. It has a broad base along the parietal bone which appears thickened. There is uniform enhancement of the mass postcontrast. What is the likely diagnosis?

A Arachnoid cyst

B Colloid cyst

C Middle cerebral artery aneurysm

D Meningioma

E Metastasis

Answer on page 391

QUESTION 57

A 53-year-old woman is referred for an ultrasound by her GP as she has a lump in her right cheek which has grown slowly over a period of 8-10 months. Ultrasound demonstrates a multiloculated, predominantly hypoechoic mass in the right parotid gland. She goes on to have an MRI which confirms a well-defined multiloculated mass. It is of low signal on T1w images and high signal on T2w images. What is the most likely diagnosis?

A Adenoid cystic carcinoma

B Lipoma

C Lymphoma

D Pleomorphic adenoma

E Warthin's tumour

Answer on page 391

QUESTION 58

An 18-year-old HIV-positive man is admitted to hospital with headaches, drowsiness and increasing confusion. A CT head reveals dilatation of the ventricles, hyperdensity of the basal cisterns and several small isodense and hypodense lesions at the corticomedullary junction. Postcontrast images show enhancement of the basal cisterns and ring enhancement of the corticomedullary lesions. What is the most likely diagnosis?

A Cryptococcosis

B Leptomeningeal metastases

C Sarcoidosis

D Toxoplasmosis

E Tuberculosis

Answer on page 391

QUESTION 59

A 3-year-old child with scoliosis attends for an MRI of the spine. The sagittal images show apparent thinning of the lower thoracic spinal cord and abnormal signal within the cord. Axial images show that the cord returns normal signal and is split in two over the length of two vertebral bodies, with a cleft of CSF between the two hemicords. Which of the following may be associated with these findings?

A Atrophy of the filum terminale

B Bifid vertebrae

C Descent of the cerebellar tonsils below the foramen magnum

D High conus medullaris

E Narrowing of the interpedicular distance

Answer on page 391

QUESTION 60

A 51-year-old man presents with painless swelling of the left eye and is found to have left-sided proptosis on clinical examination. MRI demonstrates low T1 signal and high T2 signal in the left lacrimal gland and superior rectus muscle. These areas display enhancement following contrast administration. The bony orbit appears normal. What is the most likely diagnosis?

A Capillary haemangioma

B Cavernous haemangioma

C Graves' disease

D Lymphoma

E Metastasis

Answer on page 392

QUESTION 61

A 7-year-old boy with deafness and a low hairline has cervical spine radiographs to investigate limited neck movements. These show fusion of the vertebral bodies and posterior elements of C2, C3 and C4. On review of his previous imaging, there is a left shoulder radiograph which shows elevation and rotation of the scapula. Which of the following is the most likely diagnosis?

A Klippel-Feil syndrome

B Madelung deformity

C Morquio disease

D Swyer-James syndrome

E Turner's syndrome

Answer on page 392

QUESTION 62

A 38-year-old woman presents to her GP with constipation, tiredness and menorrhagia. On examination, she is found to have a goitre. A neck ultrasound reveals an enlarged thyroid gland with a diffusely heterogeneous echotexture. There is heterogeneous patchy uptake throughout the gland on thyroid scintigraphy. What is the most likely diagnosis?

A Graves' disease

B Hashimoto's thyroiditis

C Multifocal papillary thyroid cancer

D Subacute thyroiditis

E Toxic multinodular goitre

Answer on page 392

QUESTION 63

A 48-year-old woman presents to her GP with frontal headaches and is found to have a right 6th nerve palsy. An MRI brain reveals a large mass at the skull base with destruction of the clivus and invasion of the right cavernous sinus. The mass is of mixed signal on both T1w and T2w images and there is irregular enhancement of the mass postcontrast. Which one of the following is the most likely diagnosis?

A Chordoma

B Ependymoma

C Glomus jugulare

D Meningioma

E Plasmacytoma

Answer on page 392

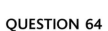

QUESTION 64

A 44-year-old man is referred for a CT head to investigate headaches. This shows a hyperdense focus in the right parietal lobe containing speckled calcification. Minor patchy enhancement is seen postcontrast. An MRI brain is performed to characterise the lesion further. The lesion is of high signal on both T1w and T2w images but has a very low signal rim. What is the most likely diagnosis?

A Capillary telangiectasia

B Cavernous angioma

C Cerebral arteriovenous malformation

D Developmental venous anomaly

E Sturge-Weber syndrome

Answer on page 393

QUESTION 65

A 41-year-old HIV-positive man undergoes an MRI brain to investigate headaches, fever and confusion. This shows multiple foci in the basal ganglia and brainstem which are of low signal on T1w and high signal on T2w images. There is no significant associated oedema and no enhancement is seen postcontrast. What is the most likely diagnosis?

A Cryptococcosis

B Cytomegalovirus infection

C HIV encephalopathy

D Lymphoma

E Progressive multifocal leukoencephalopathy

Answer on page 393

QUESTION 66

A 38-year-old woman presents with unilateral right-sided proptosis. CT of the orbits shows an increase in the volume of retro-orbital fat with subtle hyperdensity. Which one of the following additional features suggests a diagnosis of orbital pseudotumour rather than Graves' disease?

A Destruction of the medial wall of the bony orbit

B Enlargement and enhancement of the inferior rectus muscle

C Enlargement and enhancement of the inferior rectus muscle and its tendinous insertion

D Involvement of the inferior and medial rectus muscles bilaterally

E Unilateral exophthalmos

Answer on page 393

QUESTION 67

A 36-year-old man with a history of asthma and hay fever presents with loss of smell and recurrent headaches. CT of the paranasal sinuses shows several rounded masses in the maxillary sinuses and nasal cavity with enlargement of the ostia of the maxillary antra bilaterally. The bones appear normal. What is the most likely diagnosis?

A Inverting papillomas

B Mucocoeles

C Nasal granulomas

D Nasal polyps

E Squamous carcinoma

Answer on page 393

QUESTION 68

A 31-year-old woman presents with a painless swelling over the left side of her face. A facial radiograph shows a large, multiloculated, lucent lesion arising from the ramus of the mandible. CT confirms a large expansile mass which is corticated, has a soft tissue component and does not contain fluid levels. What is the most likely diagnosis?

A Ameloblastoma

B Aneurysmal bone cyst

C Fibrous dysplasia

D Odontogenic myxoma

E Stafne's bone cyst

Answer on page 394

QUESTION 69

A 62-year-old man is admitted following a seizure. He gives a history of pulsatile left-sided tinnitus for 6 weeks, having undergone a left craniotomy for resection of a meningioma 4 months ago. The neurosurgeons are concerned he may have a dural arteriovenous fistula. Which one of the following investigations would be most appropriate to confirm or refute this?

A Conventional MR angiography

B Conventional MR venography

C CT angiography

D Intra-arterial catheter angiography

E Skull radiograph

Answer on page 394

QUESTION 70

A 40-year-old woman is known to be HIV positive with a CD4 count of 45 cells/μL. She presents with progressive weakness in both legs over a period of weeks. Her family report that she has been unsteady and that her speech has been slurred. Her mini mental test score is 21/30. Which one of the following radiological findings is most likely?

A Asymmetrical high signal foci on T2w images in the basal ganglia

B Asymmetrical high signal in the parieto-occipital regions on T2w images with effacement of the occipital horns of the lateral ventricles

C Asymmetrical high signal in the parieto-occipital regions on T2w images with no mass effect

D High T2 signal overlying the left parietal-occipital cortex and causing effacement of the left lateral ventricle and midline shift to the right

E Symmetrical high signal in the periventricular regions on T2w images with further small foci of high signal within the subcortical white matter

Answer on page 394

QUESTION 71

A 53-year-old woman who was previously well is admitted following a sudden onset of severe headache and photophobia. Her GCS at the time of admission is 13. She has a CT head which demonstrates high attenuation in the right Sylvian fissure, basal cisterns and the occipital horns of both lateral ventricles. There is also hydrocephalus. What is the most likely finding at cerebral angiography?

A Basilar tip aneurysm

B Right anterior cerebral artery aneurysm

C Right carotid artery dissection

D Right middle cerebral artery aneurysm

E Right parietal arteriovenous malformation

Answer on page 394

QUESTION 72

A 4-year-old boy is admitted via the GP with a 2-week history of headaches, nausea and vomiting. He is ataxic and the suspected clinical diagnosis is medulloblastoma. Which one of the following radiological findings would support this diagnosis?

A Hyperdense cerebellar mass in the midline with heterogeneous enhancement

B Hyperdense mass in the pons with homogeneous enhancement

C Isodense left cerebellar mass with a small cystic component

D Large non-enhancing midline cerebellar cyst

E Mixed cystic and solid suprasellar mass with calcification

Answer on page 395

QUESTION 73

A 23-year-old man presents with right-sided proptosis. His visual acuity is normal. CT reveals a well-defined, hyperdense mass posterior to the globe which spares the orbital apex. The medial and lateral orbital walls are moulded around the mass but there is no evidence of bony destruction. What is the most likely diagnosis?

A Capillary haemangioma

B Cavernous haemangioma

C Ocular metastasis

D Optic nerve glioma

E Orbital pseudotumour

Answer on page 395

QUESTION 74

A 48-year-old woman presents to her GP with a midline neck mass which has been growing slowly over many months. On examination, she has a well-defined lump in the suprasternal notch and she is referred for an ultrasound. This shows a predominantly cystic lesion with some internal echoes. There is also a single echogenic focus within the lesion which has dense posterior acoustic shadowing. What is the most likely diagnosis?

A Dermoid cyst

B Epidermoid cyst

C Haemorrhagic thyroid nodule

D Ranula

E Thymic cyst

Answer on page 395

QUESTION 75

A 72-year-old man presents with increasing leg weakness and incontinence. There is a past medical history of previous TB of the spine. An MRI of the lumbar spine shows a tapered appearance of the lower end of the subarachnoid space and the thecal sac appears empty but thick-walled. Which one of the following is the most likely diagnosis?

A Arachnoiditis

B Discitis

C Dural arteriovenous malformation

D Epidural abscess

E Spinal sarcoidosis

Answer on page 395

QUESTION 76

A 59-year-old man presents with conductive hearing loss on the right side. CT reveals a non-enhancing mass in the middle ear which is suspicious for an acquired cholesteatoma. Which one of the following is a well recognised complication of this condition?

A Ankylosis of the ossicular chain

B Erosion of the lateral semicircular canal

C Middle ear effusion

D Opacification of the mastoid air cells

E Osteomyelitis of the temporal bone

Answer on page 396

QUESTION 77

A 45-year-old woman presents with a history of tingling in her right leg, painful eye movements and fatigue. Her symptoms tend to last for a few days/weeks and then resolve for some time before returning. Which of the following is the most likely finding on MRI?

A Dural thickening and multiple small meningeal masses

B High signal on T2w images in the periventricular white matter especially around the frontal horns of the lateral ventricles and in the basal ganglia

C Multiple large irregular lesions of high T2 signal in the subcortical white matter, brainstem and cerebellum

D Ovoid lesions of high T2 signal in the periventricular white matter orientated parallel to the lateral ventricles

E Ovoid lesions of high T2 signal in the periventricular white matter orientated perpendicular to the lateral ventricles

Answer on page 396

QUESTION 78

A patient has an orbital CT which shows a hyperdense intra- and extraconal mass containing multiple calcified phleboliths. The mass displays heterogeneous enhancement. What is the likely diagnosis?

A Optic nerve meningioma

B Orbital varix

C Pseudotumour

D Retinoblastoma

E Rhabdomyosarcoma

Answer on page 396

QUESTION 79

A 37-year-old woman is involved in a road traffic accident and sustains a severe head injury. Her CT head shows acute blood within the extradural, subdural and subarachnoid spaces. Which one of the following statements is true regarding extradural haematomas?

A They are crescentic in shape.

B They are commonest in the temporoparietal region.

C They are rarely associated with a skull fracture.

D They are usually due to laceration of the middle cerebral artery.

E They commonly cross the cranial sutures.

Answer on page 396

QUESTION 80

An 18-month-old boy with multiple skin lesions, developmental delay and seizures has an MRI of the brain. This demonstrates several small subependymal nodules that are isointense to white matter on T2w images and project into the lateral ventricles. There is also a small, well-demarcated mass at the foramen of Monro which is hyperintense on T2w images and displays uniform enhancement. What is the most likely underlying diagnosis?

A Neurocutaneous melanosis
B Medulloblastoma
C Neurofibromatosis type 1
D Neurofibromatosis type 2
E Tuberous sclerosis

Answer on page 397

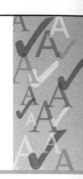

Central Nervous and Head & Neck

ANSWERS

QUESTION 1

ANSWER: D

Involvement of the tendinous insertions, as well as the muscle bellies, is highly suggestive of orbital pseudotumour.

Reference: *Grainger & Allison's* 5e, p 1398.

QUESTION 2

ANSWER: E

Reference: *Grainger & Allison's* 5e, pp 1327–1334.

QUESTION 3

ANSWER: D

This is a typical history of a patient with venous sinus thrombosis.
The commonest site is the superior sagittal sinus and this can lead to venous infarcts which affect the parasagittal areas and do not conform to arterial territories.

Reference: *Grainger & Allison's* 5e, pp 1305–1306.

QUESTION 4

ANSWER: C

The clinical details are highly suggestive of herpes simplex encephalitis, which often follows a nonspecific viral infection. CT may be normal in the first 3–5 days.

Reference: *Grainger & Allison's* 5e, p 1329.

QUESTION 5

ANSWER: D

Reference: *Grainger & Allison's* 5e, pp 1663–1666.

QUESTION 6

ANSWER: A

Epidermoid cysts appear bright on diffusion-weighted imaging due to markedly restricted water diffusion. There is free diffusion of water within arachnoid cysts; therefore, diffusion weighted imaging is very useful to distinguish between the two.

Reference: *Grainger & Allison's* 5e, p 1287.

QUESTION 7

ANSWER: C

A control film should be performed initially. Up to 2 mL contrast (high or low osmolar) is injected before further images are taken. The procedure is contraindicated in acute infection or inflammation. Pain, duct rupture and infection are recognised complications.

Reference: Chapman S, Nakielny R. *A Guide to Radiological Procedures*, 4th edition (Edinburgh: Saunders, 2003), pp 331–333.

QUESTION 8

ANSWER: B

A nasal mass with widening of the pterygopalatine fissure is pathognomonic of juvenile angiofibroma.

Reference: *Grainger & Allison's* 5e, pp 1419, 1421.

QUESTION 9

ANSWER: A

Intracranial haemorrhage (particularly multifocal peripheral or lobar haemorrhages) in an elderly normotensive patient is suggestive of amyloid angiopathy.

Reference: *Grainger & Allison's* 5e, p 1316.

QUESTION 10

ANSWER: B

The Dandy-Walker malformation describes variable hypoplasia of the cerebellar vermis and a large cystic collection which is continuous with the fourth ventricle in the posterior fossa.

Reference: *Grainger & Allison's* 5e, pp 1655–1658.

QUESTION 11

ANSWER: E

This is a highly malignant tumour which is most common in 2–5 year olds.

References: *Grainger & Allison's* 5e, p 1405.
Chapman S, Nakielny R. *Aids to Radiological Differential Diagnosis*, 5th edition (Edinburgh: Saunders, 2003), pp 251–252.

QUESTION 12

ANSWER: C

This is a characteristic appearance of metastatic scirrhous breast carcinoma.

Reference: *Grainger & Allison's* 5e, p 1406.

QUESTION 13

ANSWER: C

Spinal meningiomas tend not to cause hyperostosis, unlike intracranial meningiomas, and the majority are thoracic.

Reference: *Grainger & Allison's* 5e, pp 1380–1382.

QUESTION 14

ANSWER: C

Ninety-five per cent of branchial cleft anomalies arise from the remnants of the second branchial apparatus. Second branchial cleft cysts lie superficial to the common carotid artery and internal jugular vein, posterior to the submandibular gland and along the medial and anterior margin of the submandibular gland. If uninfected, the majority appear as simple cysts although they may have internal echoes due to proteinaceous content. If complicated by infection or inflammation they are thick-walled, ill-defined and heterogeneous. In this case they are difficult to distinguish from metastatic lymph nodes and fine needle aspiration is indicated.

Reference: Wong KT, Lee YY, King AD, et al. Imaging of cystic or cyst-like neck masses. *Clin Radiol* 2008;63:613–622.

QUESTION 15

ANSWER: D

Enhancement involving the optic apparatus, floor of the third ventricle and pituitary infundibulum is particularly suggestive of sarcoidosis.

References: *Grainger & Allison's* 5e, p 1338.
Chapman & Nakielny, *Aids to Radiological Differential Diagnosis*, p 290.

QUESTION 16

ANSWER: A

Multiple maxillofacial osteomas are a feature of familial adenomatous polyposis (or Gardner's syndrome). They precede the colonic polyposis.

Reference: *Grainger & Allison's* 5e, p 1441.

QUESTION 17

ANSWER: C

These are the expected findings in spinal cord infarction and this clinical history is typical.

Reference: *Grainger & Allison's* 5e, p 1389.

QUESTION 18

ANSWER: A

Reference: *Grainger & Allison's* 5e, p 1453.

QUESTION 19

ANSWER: A

Diffuse axonal injury occurs in shearing injuries as a result of sudden rotation, acceleration or deceleration. Typical findings include high attenuation on CT at the corticomedullary junction and in the corpus callosum, internal capsule and brainstem due to microvascular haemorrhages. However, CT may be normal and MRI (especially gradient echo sequences) is more sensitive. Cerebral atrophy is a late feature.

References: *Grainger & Allison's* 5e, p 1345.
Chapman & Nakielny, *Aids to Radiological Differential Diagnosis*, pp 271–272.

QUESTION 20

ANSWER: C

Ependymomas are usually intraventricular. The myxopapillary type tends to occur in the region of the filum terminale in young adults.

Reference: *Grainger & Allison's* 5e, pp 1283, 1382.

QUESTION 21

ANSWER: E

Asymmetrical temporal (and sometimes frontal) lobe atrophy is typical of Pick's disease.

Reference: *Grainger & Allison's* 5e, pp 1350–1351.

QUESTION 22

ANSWER: C

Pyogenic brain abscesses usually arise by direct infection, penetrating trauma or haematogenous spread. In this case there is evidence of sinusitis which has led to direct intracranial spread.

Reference: *Grainger & Allison's* 5e, pp 1325–1327.

QUESTION 23

ANSWER: A

CT is the best initial investigation as it is sensitive to calcification in retinoblastoma. If there is calcification within an ocular mass in a child under 3 years of age, it is considered to be retinoblastoma until proven otherwise.

Reference: *Grainger & Allison's* 5e, p 1396.

QUESTION 24

ANSWER: C

This is a typical history of acute on chronic subdural haemorrhage. Option A describes subarachnoid blood, B describes an acute subdural haemorrhage, D describes an extradural haemorrhage and E describes cerebral contusions.

Reference: *Grainger & Allison's* 5e, pp 1343–1345.

QUESTION 25

ANSWER: A

This is the most common leukodystrophy of children. Demyelination begins in the posterior central white matter and progresses to the corticospinal tracts and visual and auditory pathways. The leading edge shows enhancement due to active inflammation.

Reference: *Grainger & Allison's* 5e, pp 1671–1673.

QUESTION 26

ANSWER: B

The typical appearance of a parathyroid adenoma is a well-defined oval hypoechoic or anechoic mass posterior to the thyroid gland.

Reference: *Grainger & Allison's* 5e, p 1716.

QUESTION 27

ANSWER: A

Chiari I may be acquired under conditions with raised intracranial pressure, decreased intraspinal pressure or decreased posterior fossa volume. Hydrocephalus and elongation of the medulla may be features but these are also seen in Chiari II. Myelomeningocoele and tectal beaking are features of Chiari II.

Reference: *Grainger & Allison's* 5e, pp 1369–1370, 1657–1658.

QUESTION 28

ANSWER: A

Cerebral CMV infection usually presents as encephalitis, ventriculitis, infarcts or meningitis. The typical sites for encephalitis are the brainstem and periventricular white matter. Cryptococcus usually causes a meningitis which is poorly seen on imaging. HIV encephalitis manifests as demyelination and gliosis characteristically in the centrum semiovale. Toxoplasmosis is characterised by ring-enhancing lesions at the corticomedullary junction and in the basal ganglia and thalamus. Lastly, tuberculosis causes multiple granulomata (initially hypodense on CT with little enhancement but subsequently calcify following treatment) and leptomeningeal disease.

Reference: Offiah CE, Turnbull IW. The imaging appearances of intracranial CSF infections in adult HIV and AIDS patients. *Clin Radiol* 2006;61:383–401.

QUESTION 29

ANSWER: E

Neurinomas and meningiomas are the commonest intradural extramedullary tumours. Neurinomas may occur at any level whereas meningiomas tend to be thoracic and are very rare in the lumbar spine.

Reference: *Grainger & Allison's* 5e, pp 1380–1382.

QUESTION 30

ANSWER: B

Pineal and suprasellar germ cell tumours may be synchronous and if so are pathognomonic. Teratomas tend to be more heterogeneous.

Reference: *Grainger & Allison's* 5e, pp 1682–1683.

QUESTION 31

ANSWER: D

This is osmotic myelinolysis (also known as central pontine myelinolysis).

Reference: *Grainger & Allison's* 5e, p 1337.

QUESTION 32

ANSWER: E

Synovial cysts may be solid with cartilaginous or myxomatous components.

Reference: *Grainger & Allison's* 5e, p 1376.

QUESTION 33

ANSWER: B

In the subacute phase of cerebral infarction there is disruption of the blood–brain barrier and structural breakdown leading to oedema. Contrast enhancement is seen on MRI in almost all cases by the end of the first week and a gyriform pattern is most characteristic.

Reference: *Grainger & Allison's* 5e, pp 1296–1299.

QUESTION 34

ANSWER: A

Arachnoid cysts are commonly an incidental finding. They do not calcify or enhance and they show identical imaging characteristics to CSF.

Reference: *Grainger & Allison's* 5e, pp 1287, 1710.

QUESTION 35

ANSWER: B

Reference: *Grainger & Allison's* 5e, p 1394.

QUESTION 36

ANSWER: C

It is not possible to reliably differentiate between pyogenic and tuberculous spondylitis but some features may be helpful. Pyogenic infection tends to be rapidly progressive, whereas tuberculous infection is more insidious.

In pyogenic infection there is a marked sclerotic response; bridging of affected vertebrae is an early sign but vertebral collapse and paravertebral abscesses are not prominent features. In tuberculous infection a large paravertebral abscess (which may contain calcification) is a more common finding and there is typically marked vertebral body collapse but less bony sclerosis.

Reference: Chapman & Nakielny, *Aids to Radiological Differential Diagnosis*, p 48.

QUESTION 37

ANSWER: B

The low signal areas within the mass are due to flow voids as glomus tumours are highly vascular.

Reference: *Grainger & Allison's* 5e, pp 1288–1289, 1413.

QUESTION 38

ANSWER: A

Reference: *Grainger & Allison's* 5e, pp 1663–1666.

QUESTION 39

ANSWER: E

Optic nerve meningiomas typically cause tubular thickening of the nerve as opposed to the fusiform thickening seen in gliomas.

Reference: *Grainger & Allison's* 5e, p 1401.

QUESTION 40

ANSWER: E

This is Gorlin-Goltz syndrome, in which there are multiple odontogenic keratocysts.

Reference: *Grainger & Allison's* 5e, pp 1435–1437.

QUESTION 41

ANSWER: C

Haemangioblastoma is the commonest primary intra-axial tumour below the tentorium cerebelli in adults. Pilocytic astrocytomas have a similar appearance but are rare in adults.

Reference: *Grainger & Allison's* 5e, pp 1275, 1276, 1680.

QUESTION 42

ANSWER: E

Thyroid cancers tend to be cold on scintigraphy. Papillary carcinoma is the commonest thyroid tumour (50–80%) and spreads early to local lymph nodes.

Reference: *Grainger & Allison's* 5e, pp 1712–1713.

QUESTION 43

ANSWER: A

The main differential diagnosis would be a Rathke's cleft cyst but this would not show enhancement or calcification (calcification is more common in childhood craniopharyngiomas).

Reference: *Grainger & Allison's* 5e, pp 1708–1709.

QUESTION 44

ANSWER: E

Reference: *Grainger & Allison's* 5e, pp 1286–1287, 1412.

QUESTION 45

ANSWER: B

Reference: *Grainger & Allison's* 5e, p 1447.

QUESTION 46

ANSWER: B

This describes the appearances of intracellular methaemoglobin. MR signal characteristics of intracerebral haemorrhage are predictable and are therefore a common exam topic.

Reference: *Grainger & Allison's* 5e, p 1317.

QUESTION 47

ANSWER: E

Reference: *Grainger & Allison's* 5e, p 1396.

QUESTION 48

ANSWER: C

Reference: *Grainger & Allison's* 5e, pp 1299–1302.

QUESTION 49

ANSWER: A

The clinical history describes Sturge-Weber syndrome. The imaging findings include leptomeningeal angiomas on the same side as the facial port wine stain.

Reference: *Grainger & Allison's* 5e, pp 1655–1656, 1665–1666.

QUESTION 50

ANSWER: D

In an HIV-positive patient, the most important differential diagnoses are lymphoma and toxoplasmosis. Toxoplasmosis typically displays a thin rim of enhancement.

Reference: *Grainger & Allison's* 5e, p 1332.

QUESTION 51

ANSWER: E

The signal characteristics are typical of melanoma. Metastases from mucinous adenocarcinomas can have similar signal characteristics.

Reference: *Grainger & Allison's* 5e, p 1397.

QUESTION 52

ANSWER: D

The Le Fort classification applies to maxillary fractures and none of them involve the mandible.

Reference: *Grainger & Allison's* 5e, p 1443.

QUESTION 53

ANSWER: C

Reference: *Grainger & Allison's* 5e, p 1680.

QUESTION 54

ANSWER: D

References: *Grainger & Allison's* 5e, p 1717.
Chapman & Nakielny, *A Guide to Radiological Procedures*, 4th edition (Edinburgh: Saunders, 2003), pp 338–339.

QUESTION 55

ANSWER: B

Prolactinomas are the most common functioning pituitary microadenoma. They typically arise laterally in the anterior lobe of the pituitary gland.

Reference: *Grainger & Allison's* 5e, p 1290.

QUESTION 56

ANSWER: D

Reference: *Grainger & Allison's* 5e, p 1285.

QUESTION 57

ANSWER: D

Reference: *Grainger & Allison's* 5e, pp 1424, 1453.

QUESTION 58

ANSWER: E

The imaging appearance describes basal leptomeningeal involvement in CNS tuberculosis as well as the presence of tuberculomas. Sarcoidosis may have similar appearances but tuberculosis (especially with the presence of tuberculomas or abscesses) is more likely in HIV infection.

Reference: *Grainger & Allison's* 5e, pp 1327–1329, 1331–1334.

QUESTION 59

ANSWER: B

This describes diastematomyelia which has several associations, including hemivertebrae and bifid vertebrae.

Reference: *Grainger & Allison's* 5e, pp 1669–1670.

QUESTION 60

ANSWER: D

Orbital lymphoma typically presents with painless orbital swelling. It moulds to the bony orbital contours rather than causing bony destruction (although this can occur in very aggressive cases).

Reference: *Grainger & Allison's* 5e, p 1399.

QUESTION 61

ANSWER: A

Sprengel deformity of the scapula is a recognised association of Klippel-Feil syndrome.

References: *Grainger & Allison's* 5e, pp 1371, 1588.
Chapman & Nakielny, *Aids to Radiological Differential Diagnosis*, p 43.

QUESTION 62

ANSWER: B

This is an autoimmune disorder which typically shows patchy, heterogeneous uptake on thyroid scintigraphy. The thyroid gland may be normal or enlarged at ultrasound in the acute stages although it may be fibrotic and ill-defined in end-stage disease.

Reference: *Grainger & Allison's* 5e, p 1715.

QUESTION 63

ANSWER: A

The commonest site for chordomas is the spheno-occipital synchondrosis of the clivus.

Reference: *Grainger & Allison's* 5e, pp 1288–1289.

QUESTION 64

ANSWER: B

Symptomatic haemorrhage is less common in cavernous angiomas than in dural fistulae or cerebral arteriovenous malformations and it is often an incidental finding.

References: *Grainger & Allison's* 5e, p 1319.
Chapman & Nakielny, *Aids to Radiological Differential Diagnosis*, pp 267–268.

QUESTION 65

ANSWER: A

Cryptococcosis is the second commonest opportunistic CNS infection in AIDS. Early features include dilated perivascular spaces with the development of cryptococcomas as the disease progresses.

Reference: *Grainger & Allison's* 5e, pp 1333–1335.

QUESTION 66

ANSWER: C

Involvement of a single unilateral extraocular muscle and its tendinous insertion is highly suggestive of orbital pseudotumour rather than thyroid ophthalmopathy. The condition does not cause bony destruction.

Reference: *Grainger & Allison's* 5e, p 1398.

QUESTION 67

ANSWER: D

Nasal polyposis is common in adults. The polyps may cause widening of the nasal airway and/or maxillary antra.

Reference: *Grainger & Allison's* 5e, pp 1416–1419.

QUESTION 68

ANSWER: A

Ameloblastoma is the commonest odontogenic tumour. It is typically lucent and contains septa or locules, producing a 'honeycomb' appearance. It is locally aggressive and therefore requires a large excision margin.

Reference: *Grainger & Allison's* 5e, pp 1437–1439.

QUESTION 69

ANSWER: D

Conventional MR angiography and venography may be completely normal in the setting of dural arteriovenous fistula. Dynamic MR subtraction angiography may be helpful but intra-arterial angiography remains the gold standard.

References: *Grainger & Allison's* 5e, pp 1317–1318.
Chapman & Nakielny, *Aids to Radiological Differential Diagnosis*, p 267.

QUESTION 70

ANSWER: C

This is progressive multifocal leucoencephalopathy which is seen in 4–5% of patients with AIDS. It is typically parieto-occipital and does not exert mass effect.

Reference: *Grainger & Allison's* 5e, p 1334.

QUESTION 71

ANSWER: D

This patient has an acute subarachnoid haemorrhage which is most commonly due to a ruptured arterial aneurysm. The distribution of blood in this case is most typical of middle cerebral artery aneurysm rupture.

Reference: *Grainger & Allison's* 5e, pp 1312–1313.

QUESTION 72

ANSWER: A

Medulloblastoma is typically a hyperdense midline vermian mass with perilesional oedema, patchy enhancement and hydrocephalus.

Reference: *Grainger & Allison's* 5e, pp 1677–1680.

QUESTION 73

ANSWER: B

These are the most common intraorbital tumours in adults.

Reference: *Grainger & Allison's* 5e, pp 1399–1400.

QUESTION 74

ANSWER: A

Dermoid cysts are the commonest teratoma in the head and neck. This scenario describes a cyst with cellular contents as well as an osseodental structure. CT and MRI may show globules of fat with fat and/or fluid levels.

Reference: Wong KT, Lee YY, King AD, et al. Imaging of cystic or cyst-like neck masses. *Clin Radiol* 2008;63:613–622.

QUESTION 75

ANSWER: A

Arachnoiditis may be iatrogenic or may occur due to intradural infections, trauma, spinal subarachnoid haemorrhage and rarely intraspinal tumours.

Reference: *Grainger & Allison's* 5e, pp 1385–1386.

QUESTION 76

ANSWER: B

An acquired cholesteatoma is a mass of epithelial debris within the middle ear, leading to conductive hearing loss. It can result in several complications: destruction of the ossicles, destruction of the tegmen tympani causing a cerebral abscess or meningitis, labyrinthine fistula due to erosion of the lateral semicircular canal and facial paralysis secondary to facial nerve involvement.

Reference: Chapman & Nakielny, *Aids to Radiological Differential Diagnosis*, p 295.

QUESTION 77

ANSWER: E

This is a common presentation of multiple sclerosis, which typically has a relapsing-remitting course. The plaques of demyelination are characteristically orientated perpendicular to the lateral ventricles and parallel to the spinal cord.

Reference: *Grainger & Allison's* 5e, pp 1329, 1337–1338.

QUESTION 78

ANSWER: B

A varix is a dilated vein or group of veins. The usual presentation is that of intermittent proptosis which is caused by the Valsalva manoeuvre or postural change (due to an increase in intracranial pressure). Calcified phleboliths are pathognomonic if present.

Reference: Aviv RI, Miszkiel K. Orbital imaging: part 2. Intraorbital pathology. *Clin Radiol* 2005;60:288–307.

QUESTION 79

ANSWER: B

Reference: *Grainger & Allison's* 5e, p 1342.

QUESTION 80

ANSWER: E

This patient has subependymal hamartomas (which can calcify) and a giant cell astrocytoma. Other CNS features include cortical tubers.

Reference: *Grainger & Allison's* 5e, pp 1665–1666.